DEEP YOGA

Ancient Wisdom for Modern Times

Essays & Practices in Yoga & Ayurveda

by
BHAVA RAM
(Brad Willis)

2013
Revised Edition

To my wife Laura,
Who is my inspiration,
My deepest joy,
and my eternal Beloved.

Table of Contents

Foreword

Yoga and Ayurveda together show us how to achieve health, happiness, and well-being on all levels. There is little else in health or spirituality that contains such a complete understanding of the human being and the greater universe of consciousness and bliss.

Ayurveda, the traditional natural medicine of India and a sister science of Yoga, shows us how to balance our energies on a physical level, which it defines according to the three biological humors, or *doshas,* of *Vata*, *Pitta* and *Kapha*. Ayurveda teaches us the appropriate diet, herbs, life-style, and exercise for each individual constitution and our ever-changing conditions through the rhythms of time. It provides us not only with the treatment of disease but with disease prevention, techniques for improvement of our energy, and practices for rejuvenation of body, mind, and Soul.

Yoga shows us how to alleviate stress through its sophisticated set of *asanas* or Yoga postures. More importantly, Yoga shows us how to use the breath and gain more *prana*, or vital energy, both to counter diseases and to promote a better quality of energy for all aspects of life. On its deeper levels, Yoga provides the tools of concentration and meditation for bringing peace to our minds while connecting us with our higher self that is one with the entire universe.

If we can learn to employ Yoga and Ayurveda together, not only can we avoid most of the pain and disease of body and mind, but also we can reach a deeper level of spiritual happiness. Yet few Yoga teachers understand Ayurveda and how it can make Yoga more effective. They are content to teach Yoga mainly as exercise and focus on the Yoga poses only.

Bhava is one of the most dynamic teachers of Yoga and Ayurveda today. He understands how to apply them together. He teaches classes, workshops, and retreats to a wide variety of students with his own style of instruction to communicate the essence of this ancient wisdom to the modern seeker.

Bhava himself was reborn in the fire of disease, having suffered advanced cancer, which he remarkably cured himself of by the practice of Yoga alone after modern medicine had given up on him. Bhava has the wisdom from the other side, as it were, from one who is not attached to the ordinary things of this world. Yet in spite of or perhaps because of the intensity of his life and experience, there is a certain joy, wit, and humor about him. He has gone through it all and can show us what is beyond the all that we normally consider to be everything.

His book is not a textbook or an attempt to pass on any particular ideas or techniques. It is a sharing of his own transformative life-experience and the insight that he gained from it that continues to develop in his teachings. In these pages, Bhava will show you deeper dimensions of Yoga and inner healing that he himself has worked through in his own vast array of life-experience. He speaks to the subjects that matter most to all of us and are relevant whatever our background or aspirations, the main issues of health, happiness, and seeking something beyond our temporary pleasures and pains. Yet through the scope of his writings is woven the teachings of Yoga and Ayurveda and how they affect us at an individual level.

Over the years, I have gotten to know Bhava's character, demeanor and his way of expression. The global journalist has been transformed into a calm spiritual teacher, helpful friend, and compassionate guide for all who come to see him. I hope that his book draws more people to access all that he has to offer and introduces many more to the deeper wisdom of Yoga and Ayurveda.

Dr. David Frawley (Vamadeva Shastri)
Author, Teacher, Vedic Master
Director, American Institute of Vedic Studies

Introduction

Yoga can completely transform your life. Through the deepest practices of Yoga and its sister science of Ayurveda, you can maximize your healing potential, overcome great obstacles, undo inner agreements you might have about your lack of ability or power to take charge of your destiny, and make profoundly positive changes that will make you more vibrant, balanced, content, and more capable of accomplishing your greatest aspirations. More accurately, *YOU* can completely transform your life, and Yoga offers the guidance and the tools to succeed in this quest.

I know this is true because Yoga saved my life. I knew nothing about these ancient practices when I was disabled in 1993 following a broken vertebra in my lower back and a failed surgery. I spent years confined in a body brace in what should have been the prime of my life. My career as a network news foreign correspondent, every moment of which I had loved, was lost to this disability and I was in despair. I couldn't sit up in a chair to take my meals or visit with friends. My body brace spanned from my sternum to my hips, with a metal bar running down my left leg and strapped to my knee. I hobbled around with a cane. I took daily doses of prescription narcotics, muscle relaxants, and antidepressants. Still, I was in profound pain, physically tense, emotionally stressed out, and deeply depressed.

The only thing doctors could offer me beyond medications was additional surgeries. All were far riskier than the one that had already failed, and none of the surgeons could agree on which procedure was best. One specialist even suggested severing my spinal cord to end the pain and then putting me in a wheelchair as a paraplegic. Desperate, I almost chose one of these crazy options, but then came worse news.

In 1998, a series of constant colds began to plague me. Then one morning I woke up with a large lump in a lymph node on the left side of my neck. It turned out to be cancer. It had begun in my throat and metastasized to my lymphatic system. It was stage four—the worst and final stage before death. I was told there was perhaps a ten percent chance that I might live for another two years, but that death was inevitable. The lump was surgically removed and my throat was radiated. My medications were increased in dosage and strength. I was periodically mute, bloated, and became severely overweight. I became even more angry and frightened, filled with self-pity and hopelessness. Occasionally, I was dark, deranged, and delusional from all the drugs. Some people facing such a crisis quickly rise above their circumstances and become beacons of light and inspiration for others. I confess that I wasn't one of them. My inner darkness only grew deeper, and despair became my constant companion.

This darkness almost fully enveloped me when, on the brink of death, I abandoned western medicine and found Yoga and Ayurveda. It was not an easy journey for me. It took everything I had, day in and day out, for two years. With time, however, I came to understand that the challenges I faced were blessings in disguise and that most of us only find the impetus to change our ways when we are face to face with crisis.

This journey led to profound self-healing and taught me that we all have a tremendous inner power to transform ourselves. This power is embodied in the light that animates us. It is the essence of our soul. Our soul has a voice that whispers to us from the center of our hearts. It is a voice from which we have been disenfranchised by a fast-paced, stressful, and materialistic culture. Reconnecting with that inner voice, and reclaiming our inherent power, is the journey of Yoga.

Our western medical system largely views us as if we were robots, mechanical composites of interchangeable parts without an essence or spirit. It is a system fundamentally driven by a pharmaceutical industry that feeds us an endless array of pills to mask our symptoms. Most doctors are too busy to spend more than a few minutes with us, or do much beyond writing a prescription and sending us on our way. Cancer specialists rely on the "cut, burn, and poison" approach of surgery, radiation, and chemotherapy. Billions of dollars are made in this arrangement, which often seems more like a financial conspiracy than a system to promote health and well-being.

Yoga and Ayurveda take the opposite route and guide us directly into the heart and a full dialogue with the voice of the soul. They seek to balance us in body, mind, and spirit, to directly address our symptoms, and to search out the root causes and implement significant changes in our lifestyles to address these causes. These sister sciences are incredibly profound and complex, yet at the same time elegant in their logic and simplicity. While they are thousands of years old, they have never been more relevant than in these modern times in which we face so much imbalance, stress, anxiety, and illness.

My professional and personal life is now devoted to sharing the miracle of self-healing and empowerment that dwells within each one of us. It is a devotion that continues to be guided and informed by these sacred sciences. In this book, I offer inspirational essays that I hope shed light on Yoga and Ayurveda in a simple, practical, and accessible manner. Most of these essays suggest techniques and practices that you can integrate into your life in your own chosen way. These are summarized in an appendix that also contains forms for determining your Ayurvedic constitution and how you are affected by the fundamental attributes of nature.

This compilation is simple and humble by design. Since these essays were written over many months and designed to stand alone, there are recurring themes that I hope add richness rather than repetition. It has been my experience on my own healing journey that the more I anchor myself in the fundamentals of practice and reaffirm those practices every day, the more I continue heal, grow, and move forward as best as I am able.

My intention is that you will find some inspiration and some benefits—some tools to help you make the changes in your life that you desire, and some pathways to journey deeper into your being.

I suggest you go slowly, try one or two practices and integrate them into your life before trying others. This way you will create "small victories" rather than taking on too much, setting yourself up for failure, and creating more stress. Be loving and forgiving with yourself. Be strong and courageous, yet soft and peaceful. Always breathe deeply and look to your heart for guidance along the way.

I offer this collection of essays from my heart. May you fully connect with your inner light, may you heal, may you grow, and may your unique journey be an amazing adventure.

Blessings & Peace,

Bhava Ram

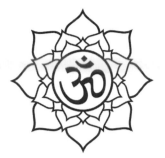

CHAPTER 1
What Is Yoga?

For most of us in the western world, Yoga is Warrior Pose, Sun Salutations, Triangle, Downward Dog...a series of challenging postures, or asanas, that we do at Yoga studios, the gym, or at home using video or audio recordings. These postures help us stretch and strengthen our muscles, build endurance, find greater balance, and take ourselves beyond our perceived physical limitations. Done on a regular basis, Yoga postures can diminish physical pain, release toxins, alleviate stress, and promote healing. No wonder millions of people around the world are becoming enthralled with Yoga. Yet many aspiring Yogis might be surprised to learn that performing these postures doesn't necessarily mean that they are practicing Yoga, which has much more to do with how we approach life off our mats than what we do on our mats.

Yoga Branding
There are branded styles of Yoga asana practice, from Ashtanga to Iyengar, Kundalini to Bikram. There's hot Yoga, power Yoga, gentle Yoga, restorative Yoga, and more, with new systems being branded all the time. We call our teaching school Deep Yoga. This, too, is a

particular approach to sharing the science of Yoga that is explored in the next chapter.

Most Yoga styles claim to be based on Hatha Yoga, which is a system of physical purification based on postures and breathing practices called pranayama, but true Hatha practices also involve a series of intense purifications that include self-induced vomiting, medicated enemas, pulling strings down the nostrils and out the mouth, swallowing knotted rags then pulling them back out the throat to cleanse the stomach, and other techniques never seen or heard of in a western Yoga studio. Hatha Yoga even holds that one must spend months, or even years, purifying the body through strict diet and intense cleansing before doing a single Yoga pose. Imagine opening a studio based on true Hatha techniques. I guarantee you soon would be closing your doors for lack of attendance! Further, Hatha is but one of dozens of approaches to, or aspects of Yoga, yet is not even considered a main path, or school, of Yoga.

Yoga of Unification

So if Yoga isn't the postures most of us think is the main practice of Yoga, what is it? In short, Yoga is the journey of you finding YOU...the bigger, deeper, more authentic, true YOU. Yoga is a Sanskrit word that means "yoking" or "unification," and it is, ultimately, a scientific, metaphysical, and spiritual practice of discovering who you really are at the level of the Soul, connecting with that deepest aspect of who you really are, and connecting with your sense of higher power, what many call God. So Yoga is both a science and a spiritual practice. Not a religious practice...a spiritual one. Yoga is fully inclusive and available to all of us no matter what our background happens to be. Everyone is welcome, be they Christian, Jew, Moslem, Buddhist, or professing no religion at all.

Yoga also means a realization that everything is unified. Everything, from the microcosm to the macrocosm of all that is. This means we are all in this together. All of us. Not just all of humankind, but all forms of life. Beyond that, we are one with Mother Earth and outwardly from there to the entire universe. That's why it's called the universe and not the multi-verse. This can be a challenging view of life to embrace, especially for those of us from western cultures that tend to emphasize the individual, foster competition, focus on the differences between us, and celebrate the ego. Yoga philosophy holds that such a worldview leads to disharmony, conflict, and suffering. A glance at world history, replete with conquests, genocide, and warfare, tends to validate this viewpoint. Yoga further holds that when we come into a state of unification with our true selves, we experience a sense of lasting contentment, inner peace, and compassion. Until we reach this stage, however, Yoga says we will suffer. America is a great example of this. We are the richest nation on Earth. We have endless freedom and incredible material abundance. Opportunities and possibilities abound for us. Our level of creature comforts is unsurpassed. Yet, collectively, we're not very happy.

Just about all of us are stressed out, anxious, fearful, angry, and emotionally agitated. We have incredible freedom to speak our minds, choose our religions, and pursue our dreams. Our refrigerators are filled with food, we are awash in material goods, we have cars, smart phones, laptops, closets filled with clothing, and on the list goes. Still, most of us are suffering. Our minds are fragmented and distracted by the pervasiveness of mass media. We are oriented towards constant consumption of material goods and yet are rarely satisfied and always seeking more. As a result, we eat too much, we drink too much, we medicate ourselves, we shop for things we don't need, we watch mass media for hours every day, we do almost anything just to escape our lives.

Depression is largely a disease of affluence, as surprising as this might sound. America's rate of depression is the highest in the world (or often tied with France); about twenty percent of the population has had depression at some point in their lives. Mexico, with far greater poverty, has less than half this rate. Americans consume more antidepressants than anyone else, and we have high rates of alcoholism, drug abuse, and suicide. The reason that we're suffering, I'd like to suggest, is that we are disconnected from the very aspect of ourselves that Yoga seeks to reconnect us with. We have been looking for fulfillment in all the wrong places. We won't ever find it in our bank accounts, the number of our possessions, our status in life, or anywhere in the external world. The only place we will find what we are really after is within ourselves. It's an inside job, and we are all after the same thing: Finding the real US.

Not only do we want better physical health, we want to live more authentically, have more vibrancy and balance, fulfill our aspirations, and manifest our fullest potential. We want to know who we really are, be connected to something larger and greater than our individuated selves, and have a sense of joy and awe in our lives. We want this at such a deep level that we are often unaware of it. All we know is that we don't feel whole or complete the way things are. This connection is the very essence of what the science of Yoga has to offer.

When we first experience Yoga practice, which for most of us is actually asana practice—doing poses on Yoga mats—most of us are immediately drawn to it. Deep within we know, even if the awareness doesn't bubble into our minds, that this is exactly what we need. It's far beyond a desire to be more flexible, have greater balance, and build strength. It's because our Souls know this is what we need, and a subtle message is being sent to us from that inner place. We just know we want more of this stuff called Yoga. While any style of asana practice can be a passageway into to deeper practices of Yoga, it's important to realize that this is only a beginning and it's not just about our bodies or the exercise. In our zeal to perform the perfect handstand or get both legs behind our heads we risk missing the incredible power of personal transformation that Yoga has to offer.

A Very Brief History of Yoga

Yoga has a multitude of aspects, addresses spirituality, philosophy, psychology, self-healing, lifestyle, nutrition, breath work, and exercise. I often call it the greatest spiritual science ever devised of how to be a human being. Yoga arose from ancient scriptures called the *Vedas*, which may be the oldest known spiritual texts on earth.

The Vedas predate the written word and are therefore more than six thousand years old.

The Vedas were divined by sages, called *rishis*, who entered states of prolonged stillness, silence, and meditation, often in the caves of the Himalaya mountain ranges in India. In these states of deeper awareness, it's said that the rishis "heard the inner voice of the Divine." They formed this wisdom into thousands of mantra verses that were subsequently passed down through the centuries in oral tradition from guru to disciple through memorization and chanting.

After the Vedas came many great spiritual epics, from the Upanishads to the Mahabharata, Bhagavad-Gita, and the Ramayana. These rich and elaborate texts are filled with adventurous stories, complex imagery, and archetypical characters that are designed to reach us at a deeper level beyond the rational mind. The deep spiritual philosophy of the Vedas is woven throughout these stories, often in very subtle and obscure ways. Yet the message is always the same at the core: Yoga is about releasing our egos and finding ourselves, aligning our lives with the rhythms, harmonies, and laws of nature, connecting with our higher power, and being better people in every aspects of our lives.

Paths of Yoga

While there are numerous different schools of Yoga and styles of Yoga asana practice, traditionally, there are four main of paths of Yoga practice:

- **Karma Yoga:** Karma Yoga is the path of action, service to others, mindfulness, humility, and remembering the oneness of all. Serving others lessons our self-centeredness, makes us more compassionate, and connects us with our deeper self.
- **Bhakti Yoga:** Bhakti Yoga is the path of devotion, emotion, love, compassion, and service to God and humankind. All actions are done in the context of remembering the Divine. Bhakti opens our hearts to miracle of being and helps us see the best in everyone.

- **Jnana Yoga:** Jnana Yoga is the path of knowledge, wisdom, introspection, and contemplation. It involves deep exploration of the nature our being by systematically exploring ourselves while setting aside our many false identities. Through Jnana Yoga we come to know ourselves on deeper levels and hear the inner wisdom of our Souls.
- **Raja Yoga:** Raja Yoga is a comprehensive method that encompasses Karma, Bhakti, and Jnana Yoga. It deals directly with encountering and transcending the thought-stream of the mind. Hatha is considered a preliminary practice to prepare us for Raja Yoga.

The Royal Path

Since it encompasses the whole of Yoga, we will focus on Raja Yoga. In Sanskrit, raja means "royal," so Raja Yoga is the "Royal Path." Approximately 2500 years ago, long after the Vedas, the Upanishads, and the spiritual epics of Yoga, came the Yoga Sutras of Patanjali. Patanjali lived approximately 2500 years ago, most likely in what is now Afghanistan. His Yoga Sutras is among the most important texts in Yoga, yet is rarely studied or taught in Yoga classes.

A sutra is like a thread, or suture, that binds things together and promotes healing. There are 196 sutras in Patanjali's teachings, yet the word asana is rarely mentioned, and only in the context of assuming a comfortable and stable seated posture for meditation. At the very beginning of the Sutras, Patanjali says that Yoga is the process of stilling the mind so that we ultimately make deeper contact with our Soul. Asana was a practice designed to make us physically capable of sitting for long periods of time in contemplation and meditation without twitching or feeling discomfort.

In the centerpiece of the Sutras, Patanjali outlines the eightfold system of Ashtanga. This is not the Ashtanga brand of Yoga mentioned earlier in this chapter, which is a form of physically challenging, vigorous asana practice. The Sanskrit word Ashtanga means Eight Limbs. These limbs offer us a scientific formula, or template, for living more consciously and ultimately transforming our lives.

The Eight Limbs of Yoga:

1. *Yamas*: Moral Precepts
Ahimsa: Nonviolence, Peacefulness
Satya: Truthfulness, Authenticity
Asteya: Non-Stealing, Contentment with What We Have
Bramacharya: Self-Restraint, Less Sensory Indulgence
Aparigraha: Non-Possessiveness

2. *Niyamas*: Personal Observances
Saucha: Purity in Body and Mind
Santosha: Contentment
Tapas: Self-Discipline
Svadhyaya: Spiritual Studies and Self-Inquiry
Ishvara Pranidhana: Constant Awareness of the Divine

3. *Asana*: Yoga Postures

4. *Pranayama*: Control and Expansion of Life Force

5. *Pratyahara*: Withdrawal of the Sense

6. *Dharana*: Single Pointed Concentration

7. *Dhyana*: Meditation

8. *Samadhi*: Absorption, Pure State of Being

These eight limbs have often been likened to a ladder that we climb to reach higher awareness. We begin by embracing moral precepts and personal observances. You might find it helpful to view the Yamas as your relationship with the world (moral precepts), and the Niyamas your relationship with yourself (personal observances). Once we do our best to live by these principles, then we purify and strengthen our bodies and minds. Finally, we unify with our very deepest self and experience our connection with all that is. Spiritual unification is the eighth limb in Patanjali's system, Samadhi. The absorption of Samadhi is an absorption in God consciousness, or the Ishvara. In this state, we have moved from connection with the temporal to a connection with the eternal. This ultimate experience of Yoga brings *Satchitananda*, or being, consciousness, and bliss.

Patanjali reminds us that it's always the journey, not the destination. Central to this viewpoint is *abhyasa*, the Sanskrit word for practice. Deep, devoted, steady daily practice over a sustained time, the Yoga Sutras advise, is the key to unlocking the shackles of mental and physical suffering, finding our inner truth, and connecting with our higher power. We must do this, Patanjali advises, with *vairagya*, which means a state of detachment as to the outcome of our efforts. This way we don't get attached to the outcome, which would only serve to make us impatient and agitated.

So why do all this? Why do the hard work to purify our bodies and minds, learn ritualized movement and breathing, meditate and cogitate, seek to move from the temporal to the eternal? The answer is surprisingly simple: it eases our suffering. Although it's thousands of years old, what Yoga has to offer is incredibly relevant for our modern age. Stress, confusion, distraction, and superficiality permeate our modern world. We feel an ever-present sense of discomfort even with our high levels of freedom, affluence, and material possessions. Despite all our medical advancements, we face a host of maladies from cancer and heart disease, to stroke, obesity and depression, which claim millions of lives every year. We feel disconnected and imbalanced, longing for more depth and meaning in our lives, more understanding of the larger picture, and a deeper connection with our true selves.

Yoga provides solutions to these maladies. It teaches us to take charge of our lives, purify our bodies, master our breath, control and soothe our turbulent minds, re-habituate ourselves, and listen to the voice of our Souls. Yoga beckons us to come into the present moment, fully accepting reality rather than reacting to it, releasing our illusions and negative habits, surrendering our egos, prejudices, judgments, attachments, and aversions. Yoga guides us into alignment with the universal principles of life, teaching us that we are neither the body nor the mind. We are consciousness…tiny drops of consciousness in the vast, cosmic ocean of Pure Consciousness that is eternal and permeates all life. At this level of self-realization, with a vibrant body, mind, and connection to our Soul, we find what most of us long for: contentment, balance, deep well being, and inner peace.

The gift of Yoga doesn't unfold overnight. It is a lifetime pursuit that requires dedication, commitment, and self-discipline. A core principle of practice is the Niyama of *tapas* mentioned earlier in the Eight Limbs, which is both self-discipline and effort, the building of an internal fire that serves to purify us. The good news is that we all have the power to build this fire and to realize the profound and lasting personal transformation that Yoga has offered humankind for thousands of years. It's not as daunting as it might seem. As I have witnessed while working with scores of students over the years, a committed Yoga practice brings incredible joy. I've seen so many beautiful people find their inner power, overcome great challenges, heal themselves in body and mind, and move towards manifesting their fullest potential.

You have this very same capacity—the same inner power, this inner guru filled with wisdom, possibility, and potential. You can move past obstacles, release old dramas, avoid new dramas, discover your most authentic self, and manifest your fullest potential. Don't ever let anyone, especially yourself, tell you otherwise. You were born with this capacity, and it is always there waiting for you, beckoning you to come home to who you truly are. Yoga is the science designed to take you on that journey, and the very fact that you have chosen to read this book means that you are already on your way.

◆ ◆ ◆ ◆ ◆ ◆ ◆ ◆ ◆ ◆

ANCIENT WISDOM
FOR
MODERN TIMES

Viveka

Viveka is discernment.

*It is paying close attention
to your experience of life,
while listening to the whisper of your soul.*

*Viveka is making decisions
that resonate at the level of Soul.*

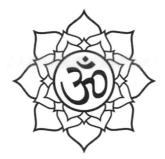

Chapter 2

What Is Deep Yoga?

Let me emphasize again that you have the power to achieve great healing, overcome obstacles, create positive new habits, transform your life, and manifest your fullest potential. This power is right there inside of you as you read these words. It's your birthright, your heritage from all humankind, your individual embodiment of that Divine power that unites us all. Yoga is the journey of unification with that power. It is a rich and complex science of how to be a human being, how to transform your life from stress and uncertainty to healing and wholeness, and how to live with greater clarity and purpose.

As I shared in the introduction to this book, Yoga literally saved my life. I was a broadcast journalist fortunate enough to work around the world, ultimately as a foreign correspondent for network news. In the peak of my career, I broke my back, had a failed surgery, and ended up disabled and confined to a body brace. I limped around with a cane to support me and I couldn't even sit up for a meal. The pain was scorching and constant, and I was pickled on pharmaceutical medications.

A few years later I was diagnosed with stage four cancer from exposure to depleted uranium in the Persian Gulf War and told I wouldn't live more than two years. That triggered a spiral into depression and despair as I became consumed by anger, fear, anxiety, and self-pity. On the brink of death, I found Yoga—the very deepest, most profound aspects of Yoga—and this is why I'm alive today. This story is detailed in my memoir, *Warrior Pose, How Yoga (Literally) Saved My Life*, but I'm mentioning it here because this healing and transformative experience provided the catalyst for the creation of Deep Yoga.

Once I found Yoga, it took me a few years of intense daily practice to heal from cancer and a failed back surgery. Along the way, my Soul let me know that my new life would be one of devotion to sharing the fullness of what Yoga has to offer. After my healing journey, I met and eventually married a wonderful woman named Laura Plumb, and together we founded the Deep Yoga School of Healing Arts (DYSHA).

Deep Yoga—The Fullness of Practice

From the very beginning, Laura and I shared a strong desire to infuse a greater awareness of what Yoga really is into to our teachings. We wanted those drawn to Yoga to know that while asanas—Yoga postures—are profoundly healing, empowering, and transformative, there is so much more to this sacred science. Yoga can guide us into finding what we all seek: A truly authentic life in which we heal, grow, own our power, live our truth, and manifest our fullest potential. By "Deep" Yoga, we mean a way of approaching Yoga based on delving deeply into the ancient texts and applying this wisdom to our lives in practical and relevant fashion. More than practicing Yoga, we invite our students to *live* Yoga, really *live* it as fully as possible in all aspects of their lives.

In Deep Yoga classes, we emphasize mastering the mind through the repetition of inner mantra and periodic audible chanting, mastering *prana*—our life force—through pranayama (breath work), and mastering the body through artful, expressive asana (Yoga poses and sequences). These three vital components are woven together to create a "meditation in motion," in both energetic and restorative Deep Yoga classes. We often share wisdom from the ancient texts at various contemplative moments in class, inviting our students to go deeper within themselves and enter a contemplative state that allows them to experience a dialogue with the voice of their Soul.

Energetic and intuitive alignment is encouraged in the poses more than any effort to achieve a precise, one-size-fits-all template for physical alignment. We all have different bone structures, levels of flexibility, muscle mass, and strength. Some of us have long legs, some of us short legs. Some of us have tight joints, others have loose joints. What feels good for one student might cause pain for another. The more we still our minds, deepen our breaths, and listen to our bodies, the more we will find our natural, intuitive, and organic alignment—with gentle and consistent guidance, of course. Through this approach, we believe practice becomes more healing, nourishing, and empowering.

The most important alignment in Deep Yoga practice, however, is alignment with the Divine. We believe our practice should be a ritual of embodying Yoga, which, you might remember, is unifying with the Soul. The experience you have on your mat of feeling more connected with your deeper self is an experience that then infuses your life off the mat, out there in the real world where all of us really need to be centered, balanced, and focused. This helps us deal with stress in new ways—to be less reactive and more present, more grounded and yet more flexible, when life hands us the inevitable challenges each of us faces every day.

Mastery of Life

Through DYSHA, we provide Mastery of Life trainings in which we train Yoga Teachers and students seeking more balance, awareness, and wellness in their lives. Mastery students learn practical techniques to open their hearts, access their inner intelligence, expand their consciousness, and liberate themselves from the stress and anxiety that permeate our modern culture. At the same time, they build their vital force while greatly enhancing their physical and emotional strength and flexibility. The journey is to heal what most needs to be heal in body and mind, knock down the mental walls we've constructed, untie emotional knots, align ourselves with the rhythms and cycles of nature, make a deeper connection with our Souls, and journey towards our fullest potential.

Yoga as Human Science

The Eight Limbs of the Yoga Sutras of Patanjali, outlined in Chapter One, are an important centerpiece of Deep Yoga practice and Mastery Trainings. The limbs are like a scientific formula for being a better human being. We cultivate a better relationship with the world and with ourselves. We make our bodies healthier, stronger, more flexible and balanced as we build our life for the greatest journey of all: the journey within. We withdraw more from the artificial, stressful, over-stimulating world around us, become more focused and contemplative, connect with our inner wisdom, and live from that more authentic place.

This said, fully living the precepts and practices of the Eight Limbs in a perfect and flawless way isn't realistic. This kind of striving can easily become a new source of stress and dissatisfaction in your life if you become self-critical and disheartened. The key is to be gentle with yourself. In Deep Yoga trainings we encourage daily practice, but urge our students to go slowly and do the best they can, never forcing things or making unreasonable demands of themselves. Small victories are always better than large failures. While it's always challenging to take charge of our lives and implement changes, the journey should be a joy, not a burden.

The Science of Life

Deep Yoga is also based on Ayurveda, the sister science of Yoga. Ayurveda is a Sanskrit term that means "Science of Life." It is perhaps the most complete and effective system of holistic medicine ever devised. Through its system of *tridosha*, Ayurveda provides insight into the predominant characteristics and tendencies of our individual natures, and how to balance and nourish ourselves based upon our particular constitution, or *dosha*.

While we all share a multiplicity of human characteristics, each of us also has a unique constitution, and in understanding this we can formulate our Yoga practice accordingly. The three *doshas* (tridosha) of Ayurveda are *Vata*, *Pitta*, and *Kapha*. They are associated with the elements of nature, Vata with air, Pitta with fire, and Kapha with earth. Briefly, Vatas are intuitive, creative, and expressive. When imbalanced, Vatas become ungrounded, lack focus, and are prone to anxiety and fear. Pittas are highly organized, logical, and natural leaders. When imbalanced, Pittas become controlling, constricted, and are prone to anger and confrontation. Kaphas are grounded, nurturing, and loving. When imbalanced, Kaphas become unmotivated, lethargic, and are prone to depression and self-centeredness.

When we understand our dosha, we have greater insight into which practices in the science of Yoga will help us achieve optimal balance in our lives. This is why our Deep Yoga Mastery Trainings include teachings on Ayurveda and guidance for students in creating nutritional, lifestyle, and yogic practices that support their uniqueness and their particular challenges in life. The is much more to the science of Ayurveda, and later in this book you will have to opportunity to determine your individual dosha.

Applying the Eight Limbs

In summary, Deep Yoga is devoted to going deeply into the ancient texts and bringing Vedic Wisdom forth in practical ways that are applicable to our modern times. We seek to share the fullness of what Yoga has to offer as a transformational science, and support our students in self-healing, cultivating greater inner awareness, and manifesting their fullest potential. While Ayurveda plays a major role in our teachings, we always emphasize the Eight Limbs as a guideline for unfolding Yoga in our lives.

To begin applying the limbs to your life, review the following list of practices based on Ashtanga, and contemplate which speak the loudest to you. What do you need to cultivate in your life right now? What might be the easiest, most doable shifts for you to make in your life right now that could create small victories? How might it be best for you to gently and consistently move forward in your journey?

Eight Limbs Practices

- Seek to be more peaceful in every way. Release negative and harmful thoughts towards yourself or others. Speak more peacefully. Walk more lightly on Mother Earth. Cultivate kindness, compassion, and forgiveness.
- Be who you really are. Drop any masks you might hide behind. Speak more authentically. Act more authentically. Live more authentically.
- Take less and give more. Choose to listen rather than speak whenever possible. Avoid gossip and meaningless conversation. Find ways to commit silent, anonymous acts of generosity.
- Tune out mass media and avoid unnecessary noise in your life. Watch less TV, much less TV. Cut down on other artificial stimuli such as Internet surfing, social media, and text messaging. Immerse yourself in nature more often. Listen to the songs she sings in the waves and the winds, the rustle of leaves in the trees, the call of the birds, the hum of all life.
- Be less attached. Your relationships, possessions, and all the roles you play in life don't define you. They all will change in time, so don't cling. Enjoy what you have but be open to the inevitable shifts. Often times, what we think is a disaster turns out to be a blessing in disguise, so go with the flow.
- You are what you eat and you are what you think, so make both as pure as possible. Eat natural, organic food. Avoid putting any altered, processed, packaged or junk food into you body. Think natural and pure thoughts. Avoid being negative or allowing others to put negative thoughts into your mind.
- Be content with your life, no matter what. Better yet, be thrilled with your life even when facing serious challenges.

Learn to smile and celebrate and affirm. Things always seem to work out better when you do.

- Create a disciplined daily practice. Even if it's just five to ten minutes each morning. Get up and do some deep breathing, a few Yoga poses, and remind yourself that you are on a journey of owning your power and living your truth.
- Contemplate who you really are at the Soul level. Reading an inspirational spiritual book often helps this process.
- See the Divine in everything. Every breath you take is a miracle. So is a sip of water, the morning breeze, a flower in bloom, a weed growing through a crack in the cement. Let yourself be in awe of all the miracles of life, especially the miracles in the mundane things we often take for granted.
- Make your body more flexible, balanced, and stronger through regular attendance at Yoga classes.
- Breathe more fully and deeply all the time. Your breath is a miracle.
- Close your eyes and bring your awareness from your brain down to your heart center a few times a day.
- Find a few minutes to just sit and be silent and still.

There is a lot here, so begin by choose one or two practices that resonate most with you. Integrate these practices into your life every day. Remember, we have to brush our teeth every day to have good oral hygiene. It takes committed, sustained daily practice to transform our lives as well. Be sure to have fun with it. Seek little victories, and then build on them. Notice any shifts in how you experience your life and in how you experience yourself. Remember any insights and epiphanies that arise, because that's your Soul talking to you, that's your inner wisdom coming to the fore, that's what Yoga is all about. The journey takes a lifetime...and it it's always taken one step at a time.

◆ ◆ ◆ ◆ ◆ ◆ ◆ ◆ ◆ ◆

ANCIENT WISDOM
FOR
MODERN TIMES

Jivanmukti

*A Jivanmukti
is a liberated being.*

*Release yourself
from the small stuff.*

*Let go of old agreements,
apprehensions, and fears.*

*Embrace life is all its glory,
its fullness, and its grace.*

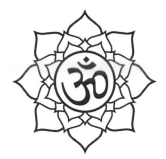

Chapter 3

Jump In All the Puddles

It had rained heavily the night before, which is rare where we live in southern California. The next morning, as the sun was peeking through billowy clouds, my four-year-old son and I set out for a walk to enjoy the clean, moist air. Before too long we came to a big, fat puddle in the middle of the sidewalk. It must have been three feet across and several inches deep. I immediately avoided the pool of water, circling carefully around one side where there was higher ground. Upon reaching the other side, I glanced back and there was my boy staring curiously at me as if he couldn't believe what I had just done.

With a wry smile he backed up a few steps, got a running start, took a huge leap, then landed—*splat!*—smack in the middle of the puddle. "Daddy," he said smiling with glee as he came up to me with his tiny sneakers and pants soaking wet, "jump in ALL the puddles!"

I suddenly understood the lesson. I had been the cautious adult, subconsciously in a state of constriction, avoiding any potential inconvenience or discomfort, and completely missing the joy of a spontaneous act. A huge smile broke out across my face as I laughed aloud and thanked my boy for waking me up. We then held hands and began skipping down the sidewalk, jumping in every puddle along the way. Soon we were wet and muddy and our ribs ached from all the laughter. It was one of the best mornings ever.

The Yoga of Expanding Your Range

If you have spent any time with young children, you likely have noticed there is something that they all have in common despite their different personalities, strengths, and weaknesses. They have unbridled spontaneity and what I call "range." They seem to get over their bumps and bruises quickly despite their initial screams of anguish. They can jump into an ocean or lake that we might call freezing, play all day under a sun we would consider sweltering, and become ecstatic in a downpour that would send us scurrying for cover. Parents often run behind their kids, covering them with sweaters for the cold, gobs of sunscreen for the heat, swathing them in hats, gloves, jackets, and an endless assortment of other items to shield them from their environment.

They are well intentioned, of course, but you might remember being a child and feeling annoyed at the endless admonishments from grownups to bundle up, be careful, slow down, back off, and watch out. It's as if we forgot what a badge of honor it is to have a nicely scuffed knee. This isn't to say that our children don't need parental guidance. It's clearly important to learn the dangers of chasing a ball into the street, riding bikes around cars, or straying too far from home. Too much sheltering and controlling, however, begins the process of narrowing our range.

As we grow up, our wings are clipped so often that we forget how to fly. We become increasingly dependent on artificially controlled environments. We turn on fans and air conditioners if it's a bit too warm, turn up heaters and gas fireplaces if it feels a bit too cool. We spend billions of dollars each year on widgets and gadgets to increase our comfort. There is a gizmo designed to make almost every chore in our lives quicker, simpler, and easier.

While there's obvious value in some of this technology, we're so awash in it that we become addicted, seeking greater and greater comforts as the natural world begins to feel unnatural and difficult for us. It's hard to imagine modern day Americans trekking across the wilderness as their ancestors did, coursing difficult terrain without roads, motorized vehicles, restaurants, and rest stops every few miles. Most of us would perish on the journey. Our culture, economy, and process of socialization furthers this phenomenon. We learn to conform, and we become fearful of taking chances, speaking out, exerting ourselves, accepting change, or trying something new. We lock our doors, set our home security alarms, and try to insure ourselves against all misfortune. The daily news thrives on triggering our fears and then commercials offer us medications and merchandise to help us cope. We begin to live our lives more vicariously, becoming spectators of life through television and movies as our spirit of adventure atrophies.

As our world becomes increasingly constricted, our lives become more mediocre, monotone, and dull. Ironically, at the same time this narrowed range gives us greater stress and agitation. When our range is wide, it contains most of life's fluctuations and we're able to accept a diversity of experiences with greater ease. As our range constricts, which typically happens as we become older and increasingly more socialized, the ups and downs of existence spike outside of our comfort zone. This causes us to respond to life's vagaries with fear, anger, frustration, and distress. With the passage of time, these negative responses become habitual, which further constricts our range, causing us to overreact more readily and to be triggered more easily.

Millions of us end up finding it so difficult to cope with the world that we rely upon painkillers and antidepressants, or seek to numb ourselves with drugs, alcohol, overeating, shopping or seeking meaningless distractions in hopes of escaping the tension that has come to characterize our existence. In this sate of consciousness, it becomes increasingly difficult for us to connect with who we truly are, to fully express ourselves, or to experience the joy of life.

Expanding Our Range

Yoga seeks to turn this paradigm around. Asana is a good beginning. Not only do Yoga postures increase our strength and flexibility while promoting healing, they're a physical expression of expanding our range. The more we can accept an intense stretch in muscles or hamstrings, master a balancing pose, or hold a challenging posture despite the burn in our thighs, the more we are also able to take more of life's aches and pains in stride. We also feel empowered, more accomplished, and more fully self-expressed as we learn to enter into more physically demanding poses. Finally mastering an unsupported headstand, for example, can shift a person's entire perspective about their ability to self-heal or take charge of their lives.

Through Pranayama (breath work) we expand the range of our breath. This, too, is healing and empowering. We become more connected with our life force and increase our inner power in the process. Through Pratyahara (withdrawal of the senses) we eliminate some of the constant noise of our society and therein reduce the frequency and intensity of the spikes in our lives. Ultimately, meditation helps us relax and let go of agitation while increasing our ability to handle tension when it does arise. Through this process, we are able to move towards finding our *Dharma*, or path in life. We can then access our inner wisdom more readily and more fully express who we truly are.

This is directly applying several aspects of the Eight Limbs of Yoga to our lives. Studying and comprehending these practices is important, but it's the doing that counts. This is difference been knowledge and wisdom. How often have you heard someone who is caught up in detrimental habits acknowledge that smoking cigarettes, drinking too much, or overeating are bad for them, yet they continue doing the very same things? How often have you found yourself in this situation? Studying and comprehending give us knowledge. Actually doing what the knowledge suggests is wisdom. You have to go beyond understanding that jumping in all the puddles is a great idea. You have to jump!

A Daily Practice

Creating or recommitting to a daily practice is an essential aspect of experiencing the power of Yoga in your life. This is the essence of turning knowledge into wisdom. If you don't already have a daily practice, consider this simple beginning:

- Commit to getting up fifteen to twenty minutes earlier in the morning. See this as a sacred time that you have set aside for personal growth and transformation.
- Find a comfortable place to sit and practice.
- Begin with a few minutes of deep breathing, drinking in life in all its fullness with every breath.
- Follow this with ten minutes of Yoga poses, doing whatever feels good and comes naturally to you, as you keep your breath deep and full.
- Finish with some affirmations such as "I am expanding my range," "I am fully living my truth" or any other positive statements that arise from your heart.
- To finish, bring your palms together at your heart center and resolve not to sweat the small stuff that comes up in your day. Then thank yourself for taking this time to heal, grow, and unfold.

During your day, look for opportunities to expand your range. It can be anything from relaxing into cooler or warmer temperatures that you typically would seek to avoid, taking stairs instead of escalators, walking or biking short distances instead of jumping in your car. Choose something new from the menu when you eat out, take a different route to work, talk to someone you've been avoiding.

You can expand your emotional range by practicing more acceptance, judging others less, or trying to force outcomes in your life. When agitation arises, as it most surely will, remind yourself that you are expanding your range, that it is already widening, and that you are capable of containing the event with a sense of calm and cool. Ask yourself how you can act skillfully rather than react to whatever the circumstances might be.

Be gentle with yourself and make little changes instead of forcing yourself to take giant steps or trying to do everything all at once. Consistency with a few things is often far more beneficial than always adding more items to your practice. You will know when you have mastered this aspect or that, and then it's time to consider your next steps. Along the way, remember that wise advice from a four-year-old child and don't miss the joy of jumping in all life's puddles.

◆ ◆ ◆ ◆ ◆ ◆ ◆ ◆ ◆ ◆

ANCIENT WISDOM
FOR
MODERN TIMES

Anjali Mudra

With my palms
pressed together at my
heart center, my hands symbolize
the flame of Spirit within,
and a prayer to the Soul.

Namaste

From the light within me,
I bow to the light within you.

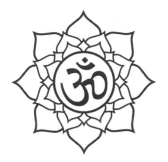

Chapter 4

The Yoga Within

Most of us feel a low level of anxiousness and discordance in the background of our daily lives. We find ourselves fidgeting and seeking meaningless distraction. We turn on the television, eat when we're not hungry, surf the Internet for nothing in particular, anything to get away from the tension. Have you ever experienced this?

Yoga calls this experience *dukkha*. Like most Sanskrit words, a simple English translation is inadequate due to the many levels of complexity inherent in this ancient language. Among other things, dukkha means suffering, imbalance, disease, despair, anguish, anxiety, irritation, uncertainty...and more.

If you feel this underlying sense of dukkha in your life, you're not alone. Dukkha permeates American culture and much of the rest of the world, especially in fast-paced First World countries. Consumer-based economies promote this inner tension because professionals of advertising and marketing have a credo: *Create a need, then fill it*. A primary technique is to cause you to feel inadequacy, tension, or fear, then offer you the "solution" to these "problems." As a result, we are awash in dukkha, rarely satisfied, and always looking for the next acquisition, adventure, or experience in hopes it will bring us that sense of happiness that perpetually eludes us. Of course, it never does.

The Art and Science of Going Within

In the Eight Limbs of Yoga, as articulated by the sage Patanjali in the Yoga Sutras, we are offered a direct antidote for dukkha called *pratyahara*. While all the limbs of Yoga offer healing from dukkha, the fifth limb of pratyahara provides an especially powerful remedy. Pratyahara is composed of two Sanskrit words, *prati* and *ahara*. *Ahara* means "food," or "anything we take into ourselves from the outside." *Prati* means "against" or "away." Hence, pratyahara is the practice withdrawing our senses from the external world to gain mastery over our minds. It is the key limb of Yoga that shifts us from external to internal practices and paves the way for inner concentration and meditation.

When we withdraw the mind from the external world and "go within," we retain our energy and expand our consciousness. This state of inner awareness and non-doing is the pathway to deep relaxation and healing. The practice of pratyahara is a central aspect of Yoga and of Ayurvedic medicine, but it is rarely taught in Yoga classes and seldom even discussed. Still, we experience it in these classes when we find ourselves more focused in a posture or fully relaxing at the end of class in savasana (corpse pose) as we lie on our mats with our eyes closed.

When our awareness is externalized, we are largely driven by our senses of sight, smell, touch, hearing, and taste. The aroma of sumptuous pastry drifts by and suddenly we are in a cafe buying a treat for ourselves. A friend suggests a movie and soon we are planning a night at the theater. A television commercial highlights a flashy new car and the next time we drive our old, beat up jalopy we find ourselves thinking it's time for a change. If we live our entire lives like this, we have surrendered ourselves to external stimuli and dukkha is the inevitable result.

Without pratyahara we cannot achieve the true goal of Yoga, which is unifying with our deeper consciousness, coming to know who we truly are at the most authentic level, and living from this place of awareness. Unless we withdraw from the agitation of our habitual thoughts and many illusions and unnecessary activities of the external world, we will continue to experience dukkha and have mental and physical pain and suffering.

Withdrawing doesn't require dropping out or crawling into a cave. It's a matter of making conscious choices about what we expose ourselves to and learning to move away from our ingrained habits of self-distraction. These habits typically include watching useless television programs, shopping when we don't really need anything in particular, comfort eating, gossiping, reading pop novels filled with sex and violence, or keeping never ending "to-do" lists. In their more severe form, habitual distractions result in alcoholism, drug abuse, gambling addictions, and binge eating. All such distractions, whether mild or severe, take us out of Yoga and lead to suffering no matter how many Yoga postures we do every day.

For instance, every time we turn on the television we surrender our minds in return for entertainment of highly questionable content and quality. We are literally providing advertisers a direct pathway into our heads. They program our subconscious with highly seductive commercials to mold us into consumers of products most of us do not need and which are often not in our best interest. The prime-time programs we watch are fraught with confrontations, violence, and ego-based behaviors. Little wonder they are called dramas. Similarly, every time we enter the company of angry, bitter, or negative people, a part of our consciousness is similarly patterned. Not only are we what we eat, we are what we choose to do, and what we allow into our precious consciousness.

The Texas Twang

In 1984, I had a direct and unforgettable experience of how subtle yet powerful the impact of our environment can be on us. I was a broadcast journalist bent on working my way up to network news. After several years with the NBC television station in Sacramento, California, I took a job as an investigative reporter in a larger market at the ABC affiliate in Dallas, Texas. Being from Los Angeles and having lived most of my life on the West Coast until then, the southern culture of Texas was a little challenging to get used to. I had to acclimatize myself to new customs, mannerisms, and social conventions to cultivate sources, conduct successful interviews, and even to make friends. One thing I avoided, of course, was trying to speak with any sort of southern accent, which would have been inauthentic, foolish, and embarrassing.

I worked in Dallas for a year and then returned to Southern California for several months before taking my next job in Boston. Soon after my return, a few friends began to tease me, saying I had a "Texas twang" in my speech. I dismissed that idea but began listening more closely to myself, and to my surprise I had to admit there was occasionally a little drawl in my words at the end of a sentence. I had never noticed any twang in my speech before it was pointed out to me, and it was hard to accept that it was true, but there it was.

As I pondering how that drawl came to be, I finally realized it was an instinctual survival mechanism embedded deeply within my subconscious designed to integrate me into the tribe. The more we mirror one another and find common ground, not just in ideology but in mannerisms as well, the more we feel connected, safe, and included. Soon after I left Texas the accent melted away and I was speaking "Californian" again.

You Are What You Think, Do, and Experience

I've recalled the 'twang experience' periodically throughout my studies of Yoga. It illustrates a fundamental and essential point of Patanjali's that we are deeply influenced by the company we keep even if we are not aware of it. Patanjali advises us to have relationships with those who are balanced and happy, compassion for the sorrowful, delight in the holy, and disregard of the unholy. This, he says, keeps us balanced, calm, and more in a state of Yoga.

Having a little southern accent was a harmless thing, but the larger point is that I was unknowingly influenced by the company I was keeping. During my healing journey from a failed back surgery and stage four cancer, I contemplated this often. I realized how negative I had become during the years that I was on heavy pharmaceutical medications and drinking too much alcohol. I realized that I had become drawn to other negative people, proving the old adage that misery loves company. I resolved to move away from those relationships as softly and compassionately as I could, and to cultivate new relationships with more conscious people whose lives had so much to teach me.

I have found in my years of teaching Vedic Wisdom that those who embark on a spiritual journey will eventually have a similar experience. As they move to a deeper place of awareness and seek to live with greater authenticity and integrity, they often realize that their "old self" cultivated some relationships that were toxic because they themselves were also toxic at the time. If they sustain these connections, they eventually realized, their old ways will sneak back and take hold again, often at an even deeper and more intractable level. This can be likened to the alcoholic who enters rehab and spends months getting sober, and then goes home and reconnects with the same old friends who are still drinking heavily. He or she is probably doomed and will soon fall off the wagon and flat on his or her face.

While we cannot control all our life experiences nor weed out every person from our life who we feel might have a negative affect us, we can be more mindful of the associations and activities we choose. We can also be more mindful of how we show up in life so that we don't drag others down with our own dramas, shortcomings, or negative opinions. I realized the truth of this as well during my healing journey, finally facing how often I had been the toxic company no one should keep.

Pratyahara Practices

Remember that pratyahara is composed of two words, *prati* and *ahara*. *Ahara* means "food," or "anything we take into ourselves from the outside." *Prati* means "against" or "away." In other words, the practice of pratyahara involves more than simply closing our eyes and withdrawing our senses in preparation for meditation. It means to mindful of what we ingest into our consciousness because it is also a form of food—subtle food that either nourishes us or poisons us. Every person we engage with, every activity we choose, and every life experience we have is a subtle form of food for the psyche that affects how we think and who we are. While the literal translation of pratyahara might be "moving away from anything we take in into ourselves from the outside," it is the practice of making conscious choices, lessening the overstimulation in our lives, and seeking to only allow in that which nourishes us on all levels.

As an exercise in pratyahara, I invite you to review your life and write down any useless distractions to which you have become deeply habituated. Is it really essential to watch all that television, listen to the radio, go shopping, or eat when you are not truly hungry? Is everything on your daily list of things to do really necessary? Review your relationships as well and determine if you are cultivating or sustaining friendships that tend to bring out the worst in you. Review yourself in the process, and be aware of the times that you may have been the person that drew your friends into negative thinking or behaviors.

Once you have assessed your life, make a resolve to move away from these behaviors relationships. Seek to cultivate the company of those who share the journey you are on, and find time to be with the teachers that inspire you. Spend more time outdoors in nature, or in creative endeavors such as music and art. Make a schedule for the activities you choose and do your best to follow it. Journal the insights that arise for you during this process, and note the changes that result from this practice.

Stillness and Silence

To go deeper, find five to ten minutes each day to sit in silence and just be with yourself. Notice your breath as you gently inhale and exhale. Notice the quality and quantity of your thoughts. Try not to buy into them and just observe the mind at work. Notice your state of being, how you feel emotionally and physically, without any judgment or concern. Do your best to slip into the present moment and stay there. Don't react to the urge to get up and get involved in the next thing.

This simple pratyahara practice paves the way towards meditation and itself can bring profound relaxation and healing. It will take time to conquer old habits, and you will feel resistance, but with commitment and gentle determination, you will succeed. Your reward will be less dukkha, decreased stress and anxiety, increased inner peace and well being, and a mind that you can truly call your own.

◆ ◆ ◆ ◆ ◆ ◆ ◆ ◆ ◆ ◆

ANCIENT WISDOM
FOR
MODERN TIMES

Sthira

Sthira is steadiness.

Sukkha

Sukkha is comfort.

*Standing in Yoga is facing all challenges
in life with great steadiness
and a sense of calmness and comfort.*

Chapter 5
The Real You

Who is the real you? How many times in your life has this inner question arisen? It's the question of the ages, right?

Who am I?

Why am I here?

What is my relationship to the world?

What does it all mean?

The practices of Yoga give us straight answers, and through them not only can we finally understand who we truly are, but also we can understand the circumstances of our lives, our interactions with others, their interactions with us, and how to shift things so that we no longer get so upset, angry, hurt, frustrated, and anxious about our lives.

You are a Divine Being.

This is an essential realization for us to make the shift that Yoga offers. When I say you are a Divine Being I am not talking religion. Whatever your religious preference, personal philosophy, or spiritual outlook happens to be, you are Divine. This is a spiritual perspective, not a religious dogma. You can be devout, skeptical, Buddhist, Baptist, Hindu, Muslim, Christian, or Jew. Please consider a few observations I would like to offer in this regard:

- No one spiritual or religious system has a monopoly on the truth.
- Some religions have been hijacked by those seeking wealth, power, and control.
- Of all the true systems and paths, none is superior to the others.
- There is a power higher than us.
- This higher power is also inside of us.
- Accessing our higher power is true spiritual practice and the key to personal transformation.

When I say you are a Divine Being, I mean that the life force within you is part of the all-knowing cosmic force that governs the entire cosmos. It brings forth life, makes the planets spin around the sun, and the galaxies whirl through the heavens. It creates and governs all laws of the universe. It's as simple as why apples hit the ground when they fall off trees, and as mysterious as the photos from the Hubble Spacecraft showing the birth of new stars in distant space. It is so deep and complex that we can only truly know an inkling of it. All our science, all the amazing breakthroughs in physics, chemistry, quantum mechanics, biology, etc., are but small insights into this amazing force.

It's the same with spiritual practice and religion. All the great epiphanies and insights in this realm are glimpses of the cosmic force. Some call it God, others Allah or Yahweh, The Tao, Mother Nature, their Higher Power, or The Divine. Whatever word you choose, you are completely connected with it. You are a living embodiment and individuated aspect of The Divine. This is why I say that you possess amazing intelligence, profound power, and eternal wisdom.

But we all forget. We get caught up in the hubbub of our daily lives and bogged down with all our concerns and concepts of how things should be. As a result, we become stressed out, dissatisfied, and frustrated. This is the primary cause of our suffering: we forget we are Divine Beings. It's likely no one ever told us in the first place, or maybe we never have experienced this awareness. Perhaps our self-image and social conditioning makes this sound absurd, sacrilegious, or irrelevant. If this is your perspective, please stick with me because this concept articulates the greatest insight into human psychology ever known to humankind which great seers and sages long have known this and sought to share it with us.

Here's how it works:

We forget that we are Divine Beings.

This causes us to identify with our egos.

This, in turn, causes us to seek that to which we are attracted.

It also causes us to seek to avoid that to which we feel adverse.

As a result, we experience deep-seated fear.

This fear creates our constant emotional turmoil and suffering.

Our Source of Suffering

A key element in the psychology of Yoga, as articulated in the Yoga Sutras of Patanjali, is the *kleshas*. The Sanskrit word *klesha* literally translates as "poison." The Five Kleshas that Patanjali speaks of, are the poisons, or afflictions, that all of face at birth and must struggle with throughout our lives. They are the reasons why we suffer, make poor decisions in our lives, and fall short of achieving our greatest aspirations. The good news is that understanding the kleshas, and implementing practices in our lives to transcend them, is a pathway to emotional wellness and self-discovery.

The Five Kleshas

Avidya: Avidya is when we forget that we are fully connected with all of life and belong to a single system, a *uni-verse*, of wholeness and oneness.

Asmita: As a result of our avidya, we overly self-identify, allowing the ego to be the primary prism through which we view the world and all experiences.

Raga: As a result of our asmita, we are constantly seeking that which we are attracted to even though these things always prove to be temporary and unsatisfying.

Dvesha: As a result of our asmita, we are constantly seeking to avoid that which we dislike even though our aversions can be limiting and illusory.

Abhinivesha: As a result of all the above kleshas, we feel a constant state of anxiety and fear that we will not be able to control our destiny.

Our Countless Movies

This process can be likened to a movie...our personal movie. When we forget who we are, we also forget that we are part of something much bigger than us alone. We forget that we are one with all that is, deeply connected, and interdependent. Once disconnected, we confuse reality with our own personal movie. In this movie, we are the star character, always casting ourselves in the lead role. We are also the Cinematographer, Director, Producer, Editor, and Script Writer of our movie.

As far as we're concerned, no one else has a movie. Our movie is all that is, and every one else is a bit actor in our script. Every scene is our creation, and it's all supposed to unfold just as we want it to, exactly the way we wrote it in our heads. In short, we are totally in our egos. It's all about us. Since it's all about us, and we are the central character, our movie is based on what we like and what we don't like. We strive like crazy to experience what we like and endlessly seek to avoid what we don't like. In every scene, we are judging everything, determining if it is in our best interest or not. We get so lost in this illusion that we become convinced that our movie is reality itself. We think our perspective is the way things are, our likes and dislikes are of paramount importance, that it's our way or the highway.

The big problem with this is that everyone else has his and her own movie going on. Their scripts are not the same as ours. Their likes and dislikes are different, and guess what? THEY are the star actors in their movies, not you! It's all about THEM, not you. Their reality is not your reality. Virtually all of us live this way, utterly lost in our own movies.

It gets even more interesting when we realize that nobody's "movie reality" is reality at all. This becomes evident when true reality comes along and doesn't jibe at all with the script we wrote in our heads. It happens in little ways all the time, which stresses us out, and it inevitably happens in bigger ways, which totally freak us out. We can't grab a bullhorn, yell "CUT" and reshoot the scene because we are not the Directors of Reality. We are merely the Directors of Our Movie, and most of the time, our script is a complete illusion.

For example, you take your beloved out to an expensive dinner at a wonderful restaurant. In your script you envision a romantic evening with a waiter who is always there when you want something, food that is perfectly suited to your taste, a meal that is served exactly when you think it should arrive, and people at the table next to you who aren't too loud or obnoxious. This might all be subconscious, and you might not even be aware that you have these expectations, but somewhere deep inside of you there is likely to be such a script tailored to your individual personality and cumulative likes and dislikes.

Then reality sneaks in and steals the scene. The waiter seems a bit rude and inattentive, the food doesn't come when you expected, the people at the table next to you are laughing and clinking their wine glasses together in a way that you find annoying and disruptive. Fear rushes through you. It's a fear that this evening is suddenly off-script, not going the way you envisioned. Your fear quickly turns into anger. You hear yourself bark at the waiter, scowl at the smiling people at the next table, then get up and storm out, vowing never to return, and ruining the whole evening and deeply embarrassing your companion.

The people at the next table may have had the time of their lives that evening, with good conversation, fine wine, a great meal, and fondness for their waiter—who was the same "bad waiter" you had! They might even have a laugh about the uptight character at the next table and say how glad they are that you left. But pity your poor date.

Man Plans and God Laughs

On this particular evening, the table that enjoyed themselves had reality conforming fairly well to their subconscious scripts. You clearly did not. They had a good time; you had a miserable time. It was the same place, same food, same waiter, but different perceptions of the evening were reached based on the inner script of each person and their reaction when all the scenes in their movie were not fulfilled.

It's entirely possibly that when the happy people departed the restaurant their scripts were disrupted and anxiety resulted. Maybe one couple found a parking ticket on their windshield or a dent on the side of their car, another returned home to find their teenage kids had a wild party and trashed the house, the third were headed to an after dinner movie and became stuck in a traffic jam that made them late. The point is, man plans and God laughs. We are not in control of reality, and the chances of it conforming to our illusions on a regular basis are highly unlikely.

Attached to our movies, we end up fluctuating between happiness and sadness depending upon how closely true reality correlates to our self-centered desires and perspectives in every circumstance we experience. This totally stresses us out. Even when things go our way and we get what we want, we begin to fear we are going to lose what we acquired. We recently received a promotion and a raise, so now we worry we might be fired in the next round of layoffs. Our stock portfolio has gone up and we are both happy and fearful of it going down. It goes down and we despair, feeling angry with the politicians, the economists, our investment advisors, and anyone else we can lay some blame on.

This stress from these constant emotional ups and downs takes a great toll on us. Stress is the root cause of the three main killers in the first world: heart disease, cancer and stroke. It's behind most other major illnesses as well, from diabetes to depression. It prompts us to make many bad choices, from eating or drinking too much in hopes of easing our emotional discomfort to becoming "shop-aholics" trying to buy happiness at the local mall. It makes us unhappy, dissatisfied, anxious, imbalanced, and sick...truly sick, in both body and mind.

The shift begins with presence. When we are fully present to a situation, and to ourselves and our habituated responses to stressful situations, we can pause, contemplate, remember our journey, and turn reaction into skillful action.

> When we remember who we really are, that we are Divine Beings, we realize it is not about our egos, our illusory movie scripts, or personal likes and dislikes.
>
> We are not the central character, pitted against the world and looking out only for our self-centered needs.
>
> As a result, we no longer react with negative emotions when things don't go our way. Instead, we cultivate SKILL IN ACTION.

Connecting with the Real You

You can relieve a great deal of the stress and anxiety in your life by remembering this system every time you find yourself reacting negatively to circumstances and experiences. Moreover, you will then make better choices and take skillful action, which leads to greater success and satisfaction.

Notice when something upsets you. Ask yourself, *'Does this arise from a desire or aversion?'* You might be surprised that it will arise from one or both almost every time.

If this is the case, ask yourself, *'Am I in my ego, thinking it's all about my movie?'* I guarantee you this will be the case every time.

Now, remember that you don't have the power to dictate what reality is. You are a part of—and fully connected to—something much, much bigger than the individual you. It has great mysteries and multiplicities beyond your comprehension. It creates ups and downs, nights and days, pain and pleasure, this and that. You cannot control it or force it to conform to your script.

You do have a choice, however, to react or act skillfully. Reacting, getting angry, frightened, indignant, shocked, furious, frustrated, or all the above, never makes things better. Usually it makes them worse. It's normal to have an initial reaction, especially given the social conditioning that influences us all, but it is immature and abnormal to cling to your reaction and allow your baser emotions to run wild.

The smart move is to realize as quickly as you can that, once again, reality has digressed from your movie script. Then you can seek to be skillful in action. Acceptance is the key. Accept that you are not the Master of the Universe and it is not all about you. Take a few deep breaths, gain your composure, and then ask yourself, *'What is my best course of action here?'* Contemplate your options and do your best.

Then, as consciously as you are able to in the moment, chart a course of skillful action. Take a chance, be open to making a mistake or experiencing an outcome different from what you anticipate or hope for. Often, you'll find what you thought was a horrible crisis was really an opportunity. The traffic jam made you turn around from your important trip and upon coming home you found your wife or husband really needed you. Even a terrible injury or life threatening disease can prove to be a blessing in disguise. It can awaken us to what is truly important in life, connect us with our inner power, and lead us into a whole new relationship with ourselves and those around us.

Accept what is.

Be skillful.

Do your best.

Remember who you really are.

Next, journal your experiences. You don't need to write down all of them. Pick the ones that really affect you, where you really felt a shift taking place. Be aware that you won't always succeed. We are creatures of habit, and habits are hard to break. Even when we know we are back in our self-centered illusions, sometimes we just can't pull off a miracle. We react. We say or do something we quickly regret. It isn't pretty, but there it is. This is okay. It happens to everyone. Even when we get really good at this, there are times *Shift* just doesn't happen.

One more thing: you might find it interesting to begin noticing when others are lost in their movies and reacting, rather than acting skillfully. It's helpful to notice this because it keeps us from buying into their drama and making things worse. Be careful, however, not to get heady about it, think you are more conscious than them, and point them out. Instead, every time you notice someone else in the throes of reaction remember all the times you have been there and have understanding, compassion, and forgiveness.

◆ ◆ ◆ ◆ ◆ ◆ ◆ ◆ ◆ ◆

ANCIENT WISDOM
FOR
MODERN TIMES

Shrada

Shrada is faith.
Have faith in yourself,
in your journey,
and in your sense of higher power.

Virya

Virya is courage.
Face all challenges with courage,
forthrightness, and a
sense of your inner power.

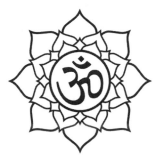

Chapter 6

Adversity Is a Blessing

Let's revisit the scene where you are at the restaurant mentioned in The Real You where you were intending to have a romantic evening with your beloved. It's the very same scenario in which you find that the waiter doesn't seem attentive enough and the people at the next table are too loud for your taste. You feel your ire rising and you are about to verbalize your anger and storm out (after paying the bill of course, yet leaving little or no tip).

Instead, you *remember*. You are a Divine Being, connected with all that is. So is your waiter and even the noisy people next to you. You realize you are back in your ego, reacting to reality intruding upon your illusory movie script of how things should go. This awareness alone is a monumental shift. Your realization prompts you to take a few deep breaths and ponder how you might best *act skillfully* rather than *react* to the situation.

During this pause, you come more fully into the present moment and notice an empty table in a corner of the restaurant that looks more romantic and private than where you are seated. You excuse yourself from your current table, find the manager, and ask if you can move. The manager is glad to accommodate you, and soon you are lost in a wonderful conversation with your beloved in a cozy new spot. Your new waiter is great, and because you are having such a lovely time, you don't even notice that your food is served later than you would usually like and it tastes delicious. The manager sends a complimentary dessert to your table to make sure you had a great evening. Driving home, you hear yourself saying, "That was a wonderful place. Let's go back there soon!"

This is skill in action. Instead of getting yourself stressed out and ruining the evening for yourself and your beloved, you worked with reality and allowed a new scenario to unfold. You softened, surrendered your ego, got over your immediate aversions and attractions, and saw a bigger picture. In doing so, you strolled off the stage of your illusory movie and stepped onto the stage of real life.

It might not always be this simple or rosy. Sometimes there won't be another table or a new waiter. Sometimes we must choose whether it's better to accept the circumstance or quietly leave, explaining that we're not comfortable where we are. Sometimes life just doesn't go as we planned and our options aren't fantastic. We get sick, we lose that which we hold dear, our plans, hopes and dreams don't unfold as we hoped no matter how much we visualized they would or how much sustained effort we brought to the process. There isn't a cozy table and friendly waiter anywhere in sight.

This is also a central aspect of making a shift:

Life is filled with ups and down, good and bad, wins and losses, achievements and setbacks.

We should enjoy our pleasures, victories, and accomplishments without being attached to recreating them or worrying about not having enough of them.

We should also face our challenges, disappointments, and setbacks with a sense of acceptance and understanding, doing our best to be skillful in our actions rather than emotional in our reactions.

There is another important aspect to this. Remember when we mentioned the old adage of being careful what we wish for? Sometimes we get what we want and soon regret that we got it. Other times, what we think in the heat of the moment is a nightmare turns out to be a blessing. It's like the story of the passenger who gets stuck in the security line at the airport and misses their flight. They become apoplectic and cause a huge scene, only to learn later that the plane they missed had a mechanical malfunction and crashed. It's an extreme example, but is has happened and the point is that we can never truly know if what we think is in our best interest will prove to be when all is said and done.

Adversity is among the greatest teachers in our lives.

We might not like it, but it's one of the fundamental principles of the universe. Most of our personal growth comes through facing challenge, pain and setbacks. Suffering forces us to dig deeply, find our inner power, and take dramatic steps to get our lives back in order. It teaches us to release our egos and accept reality, because if we remain in denial we are going to be in even deeper trouble.

It's like a piping hot kitchen stove. Universal law holds that if we stick our finger on the stove and hold it there, it's likely to burn through our skin right down to the finger bone and cause great damage. Not good, right? So, the Universe seeks to support us by sending us a helpful message: touch the hot stove and it hurts like crazy. We shouldn't be angry about getting our finger burned and kick the stove in a fit of rage, we should be grateful. We've just received a very important teaching. Touch something really hot and there's a price to pay. This is useful...really good to know.

Learn to embrace all your setbacks and sufferings as blessings...every one of them, no exceptions.

If we can make this powerful shift, we create the opportunity for great healing, personal growth, and deeper insight. As long as we're in resistance to the circumstances of our lives, we are exacerbating them. Emotional tension creates physical tension. Both of these are constrictions that inhibit our creative energies and inner power from flowing through us.

When we learn to become open to receiving, accepting, and even embracing the challenges that we face in our lives, we create physical and emotional space within us. Our power begins to flow and creative solutions present themselves. This doesn't mean that by simply embracing a serious disease or personal tragedy it will suddenly dissolve. It does mean, though, that we have enhanced our opportunity to find ways to cope with whatever we are facing, tap into our power, enhance our chances of healing, get on with our lives, and receive some important wisdom in the process.

We've already explored several principles of this process of inner revolution and it's time for a quick recap:

You have amazing capacity and potential.

True power is not an external thing; it's an inside job.

We need to make certain shifts in our lives to access our power and make it work for us.

Fortune and fame are meaningless, and even can be liabilities if we haven't done the inner work.

When we let go of outcomes and seek to live our deepest truth with authenticity and commitment, natural abundance flows our way.
Skillful action is essential, and it takes consistent effort.

This said, you are already a Master of Skillful Action in many ways.

In other words, you already have the right stuff.

You are also a Divine Being.
When we forget this we get into our egos, fixate on our
likes and dislikes, experience fear and inevitably suffer.

When we Shift this and remember who we really are,
life becomes a whole lot easier, more enjoyable and
more meaningful.

Adversity is a great teacher.

When we embrace our challenges as blessings we
create the opportunity for wonderful things to happen.

Turning Adversity into a Blessing

Within the next few hours, days, weeks, or months, something is going to happen to you that you don't expect and seems like a real disaster. It's been this way all our lives and it always will be. We are going to hope that it will be a small thing, like a broken dish, a flat tire, or a strained muscle. It might be bigger. We never know what the seismic level of the various, inevitable earthquakes in our lives will be.

Whatever it is, no matter how dramatic or traumatic, embrace it as a blessing. You might need to wait a bit until the panic subsides, so don't worry if you can't do it at first blush. Let yourself feel your initial reaction without any self-judgment. Then contemplate skill in action, determining what your best course of action might be.

If it's a broken dish, flat tire, or muscle strain the answer is easy. Don't despair that your favorite dish, the one from Great Grandma's wedding, is in pieces on the floor. Pick up the pieces and glue them back together or toss them out with a loving sigh of joy for having had the dish all those years and a prayer for Great Grandma. If it's a flat tire, fix it or call a tow truck. If it's a muscle strain, cancel your Jazzercise class and take a hot bath.

If it's a much bigger challenge, embracing it becomes much more difficult...but much more important as well. I am blessed to have the opportunity to work with many clients who have life-threatening diseases and chronic pain. One of the most important I seek to have them do is embrace their situation with gratitude. It often takes time, but when this shift happens their healing process has a far chance of being successful.

As long as we fight and resist our perceived obstacles, setbacks and challenges, the stronger and more entrenched they become. The sooner we soften, accept and thank them for whatever they have to offer us, the better off we always are. This is a deep practice of Yoga.

◆ ◆ ◆ ◆ ◆ ◆ ◆ ◆ ◆ ◆

ANCIENT WISDOM
FOR
MODERN TIMES

Ishvara

Ishvara is the Divine, God.

*When we see the Divine
within ourselves, and in all others,
we begin to feel a deep and
abiding sense of gratitude
for all that is.*

*When we see the Divine
in all things,
the miracle of life is revealed.*

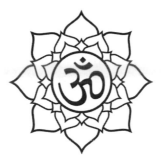

Chapter 7

Taming the Ego

Perhaps no other culture in history has celebrated the individual as much as American culture. Since the founding of our country, the archetypical American hero has been the lone individual pitted against nature for survival, conquering all adversity, and competing with everyone else for the limited spoils of the world. These heroes embody all that is believed to be good, while anything that lies outside of their simplistic ethical and territorial boundaries is portrayed as a force of evil to be vanquished at every turn.

From the adventures of Indiana Jones to the exploits of Rambo, we glorify this individual in our folklore and in our films. We have female versions as well, from Sigourney Weaver to Jennifer Lopez, with new "action heroes" waiting in the wings. Our children grow up on superheroes from Superman and Wonder Woman to The Incredibles and, like us, they are subconsciously induced to emulate their personas. As a result, often without knowing it, we become deeply "individuated," fully centered in our egos, thinking everything is always all about us.

This identification with the ego is further cultivated by defining ourselves as consumers. It is an altar at which most Americans worship, making pilgrimages to mega-malls in search of the Holy Grail, seeking happiness and fulfillment through endless cycles of acquiring and consuming. We are inundated by commercial images of gorgeous men and women wearing the right clothes and fashion accessories, driving the right cars and trucks, leading the right lifestyles, having "arrived" in their lives through the consumption of a constant stream of "new and improved" products.

We can even see the hero and the consumer in our national persona. We project our power abroad in complex situations that our leaders often see as black and white, while we consume more of the world's resources than any people in history. We find ourselves in many wars, angry that other nations do not always agree with our moral perspectives and political justifications. We also find ourselves increasingly disliked throughout the world without a clear understanding of what we have done to engender this animosity.

It is true that America and its citizens have done much good in the world, and as long as our motives and goals are honorable, there is nothing wrong with working hard to achieve them. There is a side to us that is generous, compassionate, and concerned. But over the past several decades, this aspect of our national identity has taken a back seat to aggression and greed. This egocentrism has permeated our culture and now drives our political and economic policy.

Understanding the Illusion

Yoga teaches us that when we live through the ego, under the illusion that we are the center of the world, life becomes all about what we obtain, possess, consume or conquer; and then everything seem to happen either *to* us, *for* us or *against* us, and we are destined to suffer. This theme can be traced back to ancient times and sacred texts. It is a lesson that we hear repeatedly in the Bhagavad-Gita, as Krishna admonishes the great warrior, Arjuna, who is on the battlefield of life, to rise above his ego and ignorance and slay desire.

> **III:37** *It is greedy desire and wrath, born of passion, the great evil, the sum of destruction: this is the enemy of the soul.*

III:39 *Wisdom is clouded by desire, the ever-present enemy of the wise, desire in its innumerable forms, which like a fire cannot find satisfaction.*

III:40 *Desire has found a place in man's senses and mind and reason. Through these it blinds the soul, after having overclouded wisdom.*

III:41 *Set thou, therefore, thy senses in harmony, and then slay thou sinful desire, the destroyer of vision and wisdom.*

III:42 *Know Him therefore who is above reason; and let his peace give thee peace. Be a warrior and kill desire, the powerful enemy of the soul.*

The Sanskrit word for the ego is *ahamkara*. As with most Sanskrit terms, it has a richness and complexity. Ahamkara also includes a sense of duality and separateness from others, being caught up in "I-ness," "me," and "mine." In ahamkara, we ever seek our satisfactions, brood over our sorrows, identify with our bodies, our minds, our possessions (or lack of them), our occupations, level of success, and how we are perceived. This holds us in the external world of duality and false individuation that the sages warn us inevitably leads to *dukkha*, or suffering. The proof of this is that while we Americans have the most power, wealth, creature comforts, and material goods in the history of humankind, we are among the most medicated, agitated, and unhappy people in the world.

Desire is a function of the ego. Identifying ourselves with the ego is said to cause *granthis*, or energetic knots, in our psyches and spiritual hearts. These knots must be unraveled in order for us to come to understand who we truly are. This understanding is the ultimate goal of Yoga. It involves realizing that we are not the body, mind or ego, nor are we our careers, titles, possessions, accomplishments, victories, defeats, or any external circumstances. We are eternal consciousness, the *atman* or *purusha* in yogic terms. In chapter three, verse forty-two of the Bhagavad-Gita, Krishna tells us to "know him who is above reason." He is referring to God. Later in the Gita,

Krishna explains that the divine being dwells within us, so that by "knowing him" we come to see we are much more than our individual selves and our egos. When we come to understand and live this truth, our suffering is alleviated.

Serving Others

A key practice to assist us with this process of moving from the ego to the eternal is called *seva*, or service to others. When we serve others, we begin to lose our self-centeredness and identification with the ego. We learn to stop being so consumed by our personal dramas, concerns, desires, aversions, and judgments. We experience the beauty of humility and gain insights as to the oneness of our spirits and consciousness. We enter more deeply into the brother and sisterhood of humankind.

Selfless service, of course, is not the sole purview of Yoga. Many religions and spiritual traditions embrace service as a pathway to the divine, and service clubs with no religious or spiritual affiliations exist throughout the world. In Yoga, such service is part of the practice of *Karma Yoga*, the Yoga of positive action. Practicing seva as part of Karma Yoga helps us connect with God through seeing and serving God in others. It also helps alleviate negative karma, and even helps cure diseases and prepares us for the higher states of Yoga and self-realization.

Our practice of seva can be small or it can be grand. We can help an elderly neighbor do chores around their home, or we can devote ourselves to global projects to feed the starving or promote peace. The most important part of seva is to ensure we are acting from the heart without any desire for notoriety or recognition. Wealthy people who donate large sums of money in order to have their names placed on plaques or buildings are not practicing seva. While they are being generous, they also desire to be acknowledged for their generosity, which is often due to ulterior motives of self-promotion and profit. Seva is always meant to be done with humility and without expectation of recognition. It is fine if honors and accolades come to us as a result of our work, but they should never be our goal, and we should never become enamored with such recognition, for it is yet another form of desire.

Seva also can be integrated into our livelihoods. A good friend and colleague of mine, Chris Rutgers, was on his way to being a professional skier when a broken back ended his career. Chris had been severely abused as a child, and he found that skiing and outdoor activities were keys to overcoming his emotional pain and moving on with his life. When his career as an athlete abruptly came to a halt, Chris founded a nonprofit corporation in San Diego called Outdoor Outreach to help at-risk kids overcome their circumstances and build confidence and self-esteem through a variety of group outdoor activities. As a result of this seva, Chris has turned scores of lives around and has also created a very meaningful life for himself.

We are not all going to rush out and found nonprofit agencies, but if we open our hearts to seva, it will find us. I have seen this happen in my Deep Healing classes at Ginseng Yoga Studio in San Diego. One student rides the bus to attend these evening classes. He only lives ten minutes away by car, but it usually takes more than an hour on the bus. He has a bad heart, and it's a tough trip to make every week. When I am able to, I drive him home after class. After choosing seva as our theme one evening, I asked if someone else would like to give him ride as it was not possible for me to take him home that evening. Several volunteers came forth, and now he always has transportation, not just going home, but both ways! In practicing this seva, these students are taking their Yoga up off their mats and integrating it into their lives. Through this process, they are unraveling the knots of ahamkara that we all face, opening their hearts, and moving to deeper levels of awareness.

As an experiment, open yourself to the idea of seva over the next few weeks. See what opportunities arise as a result of your openness and embrace the first one that you feel you are capable of doing. Again, it needn't be a grand gesture or long-term commitment. Just devote your heart to it and enjoy the inner reward of doing seva for no reason other than the joy of giving and the acknowledgement of the divine in all of humankind.

In doing so, you begin to "live" Yoga. The reward for such service, you will likely find, is far greater than public recognition or financial reward. It is the reward of peace and oneness that you will feel at the very core of your being.

◆ ◆ ◆ ◆ ◆ ◆ ◆ ◆ ◆ ◆

ANCIENT WISDOM
FOR
MODERN TIMES

Vidya

Vidya is wisdom.

*The eternal wisdom
that you always have been,
and always will be, one with all that is.*

*Vidya is the ultimate realization of Yoga,
a returning to source,
and finding that very source
within you.*

Chapter 8
The Alchemy of Yoga

When a broken back and failed surgery ended my career as a foreign news correspondent and left me in constant pain, I began a slow descent into darkness without even realizing it. The painkillers and tranquilizers western doctors prescribed deepened my despondency while at the same time numbed my consciousness and masked my soul. The subsequent "terminal" cancer I contracted from exposure to depleted uranium while covering the Persian Gulf War as a news correspondent plunged me into the abyss. I felt like a victim, that adversaries and enemies abounded, that the whole world was conspiring against me. As my anger and frustration increased, I alienated family and friends, my world contracted, and I moved towards despair.

Most of us have known people who always seem to live under a dark cloud. They move from crisis to crisis and are plagued by illnesses, accidents, failures, conflicts, and disappointments. Many of us also have known those special people who seem to float through life achieving their goals, manifesting their dreams, and having almost everything effortlessly go their way. It's not a matter of bad fortune for some and good luck for others, these "winners" and "losers" have created their own realities through a powerful process of inner alchemy.

Alchemy is a complex term whose etymology dates back to ancient Greek and Egypt. For some, it calls up images of primeval crackpots and charlatans promising to turn lead into gold. For others, it reminds us of the genius of Sir Isaac Newton who, as an alchemist, astronomer, naturalist, and physicist, was among of the greatest scientists and mathematicians of all times. Through exploration of alchemy, Newton delved into the metaphysical and spiritual aspects of reality.

Ancient alchemists, like their Yogi counterparts, saw all creation as composed of the five primary elements, called *mahabhutas*, of earth, air, fire, water, and space. Through their meditations and explorations of these five elements, they created healing and transformative potions that eventually formed the base of much of modern pharmacology. In the process, they unlocked many of the mysteries of the Universe and therein contributed to the evolution of humankind.

Alchemy, in the realm of metaphysics, is arguably the higher practice of this ancient art. Just as pure gold can be obtained by burning away its impurities and base metals, through spiritual alchemy one can move from an imperfect, diseased, ignorant, and corrupted state towards wisdom, healing, self-transformation, and enlightenment. This is the alchemy of Yoga.

You Are What You Think

When a bear is chasing us in the woods, we enter into an instinctive "fight or flight" response. We don't even have to think about it. Our bodies flood with adrenalin and cortisol, giving us power and energy to run as fast as possible or turn and fight for our lives. This is a very good thing whenever we are faced with truly cataclysmic events. The problem is that our fast paced, high stress culture continuously triggers this state of fight or flight even though it isn't necessary for our survival. The stress this causes hovers in the backgrounds of our daily lives and then, all too often, boils to the surface and takes over. We become quick to anger, fear, doubt, anxiousness, insecurity, and a host of other negative emotions that keep us pickled on adrenalin and cortisol. In this state, our immune system and digestive functions are placed on hold because the body wants all its energy to deal with the perceived emergency. This condition usually leads to mental and physical ailments and disease.

The thoughts of a more positive person who isn't so reactive to life create healing neuropeptides such as serotonin and acetylcholine. These chemicals boost the immune function, relax the heart rate, support digestion, and promote healing. This is the state of "rest and digest" and leads to a happier life in which we experience greater physical and emotional health, feel more balanced, and we're more skillful in living our lives.

Simply put: You are what you think. The hypochondriac becomes sick. The pessimist creates a reality in which things always seem to go wrong. Those who believe they cannot accomplish something have already seeded their own defeat. The optimist who takes a sugar pill in a blind test of a new medicine may experience benefits far beyond what the real drug has to offer. Those who are convinced of their potential are likely to realize it no matter what obstacles arise. Those who see the world filled with light and love often have this reflected back to them as their reality.

The Miraculous Case of Mr. Wright

In 1950, a patient named Mr. Wright had an extremely advanced case of cancer, with tumor masses the size of oranges in his neck, groin, chest, and abdomen. His spleen and liver were severely enlarged. His primary lymphatic duct was obstructed, and up to two liters of milky fluid had to be drawn from his chest every other day. Finally, his doctors gave him less than two weeks to live.

Then came news of an experimental drug named Krebiozen, formulated to treat this virulent type of cancer. Mr. Wright's oncologist, Doctor Bruno Klopfer, was conducting trials of the new drug, but felt his patient was too far gone to participate. Mr. Wright persisted, begging the doctor to give him one last chance for life. Dr. Klopfer finally consented, thinking at least his patient might have some comfort during his last days knowing that there was hope, be it a false hope or not.

Three days after his first injection, Mr. Wright experienced astonishing results. According to Dr. Klopfer's medical notes, "The tumor masses melted like snowballs on a hot stove, and in only a few days were half their original size."

Surprisingly, none of the other patients in the trial experienced any changes and later Krebiozen was proven useless for the treatment of cancer. Yet within ten days of his first injection, Mr. Wright was discharged from hospital, "Practically all signs of his disease having vanished." A few months later, however, reports appeared in the media that Krebiozen was ineffective. When Mr. Wright read the news he lost faith, became depressed, and soon relapsed into his former state of ill health—tumors and all.

His doctor was stunned, but viewed this as an opportunity to test the placebo effect: the ability of patients to heal based on their belief in a treatment. So Dr. Klopfer deliberately deceived Mr. Wright with a story about receiving a newly formulated "super-refined, double strength" batch of Krebiozen with great healing potential. Convinced by this ruse, Mr. Wright's faith was restored and he eagerly began a second treatment program. His new injections were nothing more than fresh water, but the results were as astounding as the first time. His tumor masses melted, his chest fluid vanished, and Mr. Wright became a picture of health, even taking up his old hobby of flying airplanes.

Mr. Wright was symptom free for over two months, until he read that the AMA had definitively declared Krebiozen a useless drug. His doubt returned and he went off the injections. Shortly thereafter, he was readmitted to the hospital in a deeply distressed condition. Two days later he was dead.

This remarkable story is documented. It was reported in 1957 by one of Mr. Wright's personal physicians, Dr. Philip West, and published in *The Journal of Projective Techniques*.

Inner Alchemy

Again, each of us is an alchemist capable of creating a host of complex elixirs, potions and drugs. Our laboratory is our brain. The formulas are created by the quality of our thoughts. Once we create them, they course throughout our neurological and cardiovascular systems and flow into our organs, muscles, bones, and tissues. As a result, we are either creating black magic that causes us pain, or we are concocting miracle potions that help us heal and lead more meaningful lives.

Negative emotions do the greatest harm to our health.

Negative emotions create stress.

Negative emotions diminish organ function.

Negative emotions decrease circulation.

Negative emotions weaken our immune system.

Negative emotions promote negative choices.

Negative thinking not only make us unhappy, it poisons us. On a physical level, it creates a biochemical toxicity that diminishes our health and overall capacity to function. On a psychological level, it diminishes our mental capacity, inhibits our ability to creatively respond to the challenges of life, and stunts our personal growth. Just as many weary soldiers return home with Post Traumatic Stress Disorder after tours of heavy combat, we are creating our own form of mini-PTSD every day. These life-or-death responses to the little irritations in our lives never promote solutions. This is why so many of us end up on tranquilizers while paying therapists to listen to our troubles.

The "fight or flight" response does have a very positive aspect. If a bear really is about to attack, our flight mechanism will take charge and we'll run faster than we believed possible. If we can't escape the bear, our fight response will empower us to resist beyond what we thought possible. Either way, it's a handy survival instinct for all animals in times of great crisis. A certain level of adrenalin can also help us be more motivated and productive in our lives, but somehow this function has gone haywire in the human species and our brains fail to discriminate between life-threatening events and insignificant ones.

The thoughts of a positive alchemist, on the other hand, create soothing chemicals that relax our adrenals, calm us in body and mind, and promote healing. This is why a positive outlook is so powerful. It creates "miracle drugs" in our brains and delivers them throughout our bodies. We don't need a prescription for this medicine and, better yet, it's completely free and has no side effects.

Positive emotions decrease stress.

Positive emotions enhance organ function.

Positive emotions increase circulation.

Positive emotions strengthen our immune systems.

Positive emotions promote positive choices.

Praying for What We Don't Want

If this is so good for us, then why is it so hard to replace negative emotions with positive ones? Why is it such a challenge to be happy? First, most of us become addicted to the drama. Second, we live in a culture designed to endlessly trigger this response. Turn on the news and you'll hear nothing but calamity. They want us to be worried about everything happening today so we'll stay tuned to find out how it all worked out. Most movies and TV dramas also glorify constant confrontation and conflict.

We learn to mirror these dramatic encounters in our own lives, patterning our behaviors and personalities on dysfunctional social behaviors created by screenwriters. Advertisers know the more we experience vicarious anger and fear, the more we'll consume things in hopes of easing our anxiety. They deliberately stir us up so we'll spend money trying to escape the agitation they offer us in the name of entertainment. Worrying is like praying for what we don't want to happen in our lives. Positive people, on the other hand, usually have better outcomes because their perspective is like a prayer for what they do want in their lives.

We can't all melt cancer tumors away with positive thoughts like Mr. Wright, but his experience provides a dramatic example that it's always an inside game. Through faith and positive attitudes we can access our inherent power to heal, often in the most challenging of circumstances. As we respond to our circumstances, experiences, and surroundings, we directly affect how they respond and reflect back to us. We are the alchemists not only of the chemicals coursing through our bodies; we are the creators of our individual worlds. This is why Yoga, and its sister science of Ayurveda, teach us alchemical techniques that reconstruct the molecules of our beings.

From Patanjali's Eight Limbs of Yoga, the fifth limb, *Pratyahara* (withdrawal of the senses), and the sixth, *Dharana* (single-pointed concentration), bring us to deeper levels of inner awareness and balance. Mantra—the repetition of sacred words—allows us to access higher universal powers that are healing and transformative. The seventh limb, *Dhyana* (meditation), ultimately crystallizes our consciousness and guides us towards self-realization. All these practices are alchemical. They change our inner chemistry, which in turn supports us in making the emotional shifts we seek in life.

Creating Your Own Healing Elixirs

As a practice, you can conduct your own scientific experiment, serving both as scientist and subject, with your brain as the laboratory. Find a quiet place where you can lie down undisturbed for several minutes (this can be done at the end of Yoga exercises laying on your back during *savasana*, or as a response to a stressful day or incident). Once you are comfortable, take note of your emotional state as you begin. Try to feel the "taste" inside of your body, the current chemical atmosphere of your being. Bring your awareness to your brain, seeing it as your laboratory and your mind as the scientific alchemist. Then, allow your breath to become deep and full. After a few breaths, begin placing the following words in your brain, silently repeating each one long enough that the emotion of the word begins to permeate your consciousness.

Contentment... Repeat this over and over with your breath remaining deep and full, really feeling it, breathing it into your heart and exhaling it throughout your entire being. Do this for a few minutes, noticing the internal chemistry of your body and the subtle shifts that begin to take place.

Serenity... Follow the same process.

Then move through the following positive emotions:

Peace... Gratitude... Compassion... Loving Kindness... Forgiveness...

Spend a few minutes with each of these emotions or any other positive feelings you feel you need. You don't have to memorize these words or this sequence. Choose the words that you know deep in your heart are the most healing and transformative for you, even letting them arise naturally during the process. You might choose courage, power, or peace...whatever resonates with you. When you're done, spend some time noticing any shifts in your inner essence, any different "taste" of being you. Feel the relaxation and pleasure that arises from this practice in every cell of your body and every corner of your mind.

This alchemical process played a major role in my own self-healing from cancer and a broken back. Once I left western medicine and embraced Yoga and Ayurveda, I learned to take responsibility for the world I was creating for myself. I moved from fear, anger, and despondency to openness, compassion, and a firm belief in my ability to self-heal. It didn't happen overnight, and at times it felt like I was endlessly digging ditches, seeking to pierce the crust of my entrenched emotions so that I might at last unearth a deeper place in my Soul where my true nature was buried. Yet through faith, devotion, and dedication, the work eventually paid off and I was fortunate enough to heal, both physically and emotionally.

Healing, I came to learn afterwards, did not stop there. It is a daily practice in a world where stressful challenges and negative emotions often prevail. We need to work at it, stay devoted to the practice, and have faith in our inherent capacity to transform our lives. We also need to cultivate patience. True healing doesn't happen overnight, it's a lifelong journey.

◆ ◆ ◆ ◆ ◆ ◆ ◆ ◆ ◆ ◆

ANCIENT WISDOM
FOR
MODERN TIMES

Moksha

Moksha is liberation
from the tyranny of our
smaller selves.

Moksha is mastering the
mind and body, expanding our life force,
and determining the course of our destiny.

Yoga is the pathway that
leads us to moksha.

Chapter 9

Know Thyself

If the ancient sages who spent years in solitude in the caves of the Himalaya Mountains were to walk into a Yoga class anywhere in America today, they likely would be surprised, and perhaps a little bewildered. Despite their great wisdom and insight, it might even take them a few minutes to realize that the students were practicing Yoga.

Traditionally, Yoga was an individual practice and not a group activity. Practitioners would seek the guidance of a guru and gather with this teacher when possible, but their Yoga was largely performed individually and focused on mantra, pranayama, meditation, and purifications such as fasting, lengthy periods of silence, and seclusion. Practices were highly individualized and often came as a result of consultations with an expert in Ayurveda, the sister science of Yoga.

Remember that Ayurveda, which translates as the science of Life, is perhaps the oldest and most complete system of holistic medicine ever devised. While it has a strong spiritual component, it was designed to purify the body and mind as a preparation for the spiritual journey of Yoga. The logic of this is that the body is the temple of our Spirit, and that impurities or imbalances in the body and mind are impediments to self-realization, which is the focal point of Yoga.

Often, one would spend months, or even years, in Ayurvedic treatment before practicing Yoga. This doesn't mean, however, that they wouldn't do any asanas, because while Yoga poses are not Yoga itself, they are essential tools of both Ayurveda and Yoga. In the Yoga Sutras, the great sage Patanjali seems to allude to this in the very first verse, or Sutra:

Sutra I:1 *Atha Yoganusasanam.*
Now, the instruction of Yoga.

Some Vedic scholars hold that this simple introductory sutra references Ayurveda with the word "now." In other words, Patanjali, who was a master of Ayurveda as well as Yoga, is assuming that the reader has already had significant exposure to Ayurveda, that body and mind have been purified and balanced to some degree, and that the aspirant is now ready for the journey into Yoga.

Through Ayurveda, the practitioner's fundamental constitution, his or her dosha, would already be determined. Unlike the four humors of traditional Greco-Roman and European Medieval medicine which were considered fluids, the doshas are manifestations of elemental forms in the physical body and not physical substances in themselves. As first mentioned in Chapter Two, Ayurveda holds that there are three doshas: Vata, Pitta, and Kapha. Vata is associated with air, Pitta with fire, and Kapha with water. Each of us possesses a mixture of all three of these doshas, but usually one is our predominant dosha. In some cases two or all three doshas are predominant, and it can become quite complex in diagnosis and treatment. One dosha is not better than another, nor is having a constitution with two or all three doshas superior. Dosha also means imbalance, and we become imbalanced and suffer when our dosha becomes excessive or deranged.

When balanced, Vatas tend to be very creative and free flowing, like the wind. They are open-minded and quickly grasp a diversity of topics. They are sensitive, good communicators, and energetic. As they become imbalanced they tend to be restless, full of desires, and never satisfied. They flit from one thing to another. Yoga this week, Tai Chi the next, then maybe some Qi Gong or some other popular practice the week after...and so forth. Then a Vata type might drop it all and dive into less conscious pursuits. Their minds become easily distracted and whirl round like a storm. When Vatas face stress and challenges, their emotional reaction is usually fear and anxiety. They can be inclined towards drugs, alcoholism, and other self-destructive indulgences and escapes. They become deceptive and erratic, and in extreme cases can be suicidal.

Balanced Pittas are warm and intelligent. They are very disciplined, receptive, and discriminating. Pittas are natural leaders, typically courageous and compassionate. They are often found in leadership positions in politics, law, and industry. As they become imbalanced, Pittas are often aggressive, willing to do whatever it takes to succeed, mowing down those who get in their way. They lust for power and wealth, are critical and controlling, and prone to ego, anger, and vanity. Pittas' response to stress and challenge is usually anger. They harbor hatred, resentment, and hostility. At their worst, Pittas can be paranoid and psychopathic.

Balanced Kaphas are filled with love, devotion, faith and contentment. They are steady, patient and deeply caring. They are also loyal, forgiving, nurturing, and supportive. People naturally feel accepted and embraced when around balanced Kaphas, but as they become imbalanced, Kaphas tend to be self-centered and like to accumulate possessions and wealth. This greed and materialism leaves them perpetually unsatisfied and ever lusting for more. Food is often Kaphas chosen form of overindulgence, and they are highly susceptible to weight gain. When Kaphas face stress and challenge they become lethargic and depressed. In this state, Kaphas refuse to make any effort and blame others for their demise.

Ayurveda seeks to bring the doshas back into balance through a variety of techniques including diet, lifestyle alterations, special herbs, purifications, Yoga poses, pranayama, mantra and meditation. Each treatment program is designed specifically for the individual and takes into account age, occupation, mental outlook, gender, physical ability, and a host of other attributes and tendencies that make each of us unique.

This is why the sages might be surprised to see a class full of Yoga students all practicing the same asanas. These classes are wonderful and offer a host of benefits, but there is no "one size fits all" in Yoga, and part of being in balance involves determining what asana program best suits our dosha. This is important because when we have an imbalance, we tend to create habits that feed it and make it worse. We'll now look at this tendency through the prism of asana.

Dosha and Yoga Classes of Choice

Remember, Vatas are like the wind and drawn to change. If you determined the doshas of the students in most free-flowing Vinyasa style classes, with varied music and no set routines, you are likely to find Vatas. Pittas like logic and control. In an exacting "Power Yoga" or strictly technical asana class you will find more Pittas. Kaphas like relaxation and indulgences that require minimum effort. A restorative or slow-paced, non-challenging class is likely to attract Kaphas. In each case, from an Ayurvedic standpoint, the students are feeding their imbalances. This is not so dangerous that they'll find themselves entering into the deeply negative emotional tendencies of their dosha as a result, but it does make balancing their dosha more difficult.

As an Ayurvedic practitioner, I would advise most Pittas to occasionally cool their fire in a more restorative class. I would recommend that Vatas try to attend more technical classes where they are required to follow set routines and hold poses for long periods of time that help to ground them. I would ask Kaphas put aside their blocks, bolster, blankets, and pillows and get into more rigorous classes that require greater effort and exertion. If these students were clients of our Deep Healing programs, the daily routines designed for them also would follow these guidelines. This doesn't mean they would be banned from ever doing the classes they feel most drawn to, but their practice would become more diversified and oriented towards balancing their dosha.

In talking about balance, imbalance, and derangement, I'm also referencing the Ayurvedic concept of the *gunas*. The gunas are the three primal forces of nature, known as *tamas, rajas* and *sattva*. Guna means "that which binds," because the gunas keep us in bondage to the external world, which therefore keeps us in a state of suffering. While the doshas are horizontal—meaning one dosha is not more desirable than another—the gunas are vertical.

At the bottom, tamas is associated with dullness, darkness, and inertia, the least desirable guna. A tamasic person, no matter their dosha, is likely to be unemployed, heavily addicted, and barely able to take care of themselves.

Rajas is associated with change, activity and turbulence. A rajasic person will be highly active, which helps lift them out of tamas, but they soon become agitated, over-stressed, and constantly caught up in doing.

Sattva is intelligence, harmony, and stability. A sattvic person has moved beyond rajas and is calmer in their actions and more satisfied with life.

Ayurveda seeks to identify where any individual is tamasic and move them towards rajas and then into sattva. A deeply tamasic person is unlikely ever to seek any help or healing. Most who come to Yoga and Ayurveda have some tamas, mostly rajas and often some sattva as well. Again, it can be complex, and we all have the tendency to shift between the gunas as our lives fluctuate and change.

Know Thyself

I've included two forms in the appendix section of this book to help you determine your dosha and to help you see where you are with the gunas. Do your best to fill the forms out quickly and intuitively without seeking a particular outcome. It is important to be deeply honest with yourself. It often helps to then have someone who knows you well, and whose judgment you value, look at your answers and give you their opinions on your characteristics.

Through these forms you will get an Ayurvedic snapshot of yourself. By knowing your dosha you can begin to consider making choices in your life that might bring it into greater balance rather than feeding your imbalances. Choosing to attend more of the right asana classes might be a beginning. By simple logic, you can also identify other activities that might not suit your dosha. For instance, a Vata might want to avoid constant change and seek activities that ground them, such as walking in nature and contemplating mountains and trees. A Pitta might avoid strenuous and competitive activities and seek to be a bit more free flowing. Oceans and rivers would be good to frequent and contemplate. A Kapha might avoid being a couch potato in favor of vigorous hikes and more strenuous activities.

By filling out and analyzing the guna form, you will begin to identify the areas in which you need to place the greatest emphasis. Look at any tamasic tendencies first and contemplate how you might best address them. If you feel you have none, look at the rajasic tendencies and choose a few to work on. Don't be in a hurry, and don't expect to move yourself fully into the sattva column overnight. Becoming sattvic is usually a lifetime pursuit. For many of us it might take several lifetimes! Be gentle with yourself and go slowly.

There is much more to this system, including specific recommendations on lifestyle, nutrition, herbology, pranayama, mantra, meditation and more. If you want to explore it further, consider having a consultation with a qualified practitioner of Ayurveda. Still, cultivating an elemental understanding of the doshas and gunas heightens your awareness, helps you to truly know yourself, and takes you deeper into the journey of Yoga.

◆ ◆ ◆ ◆ ◆ ◆ ◆ ◆ ◆ ◆

ANCIENT WISDOM
FOR
MODERN TIMES

Abhyasa

*Abhyasa is consistent practice
and full dedication to your
chose path of personal growth.*

Vairagya

*Vairagya is detachment
as to the outcome
of your practice.*

Chapter 10
Minding

One of the greatest Vedic thinkers and spiritual teachers of modern times was J. Krishnamurti (1895-1986). Krishnamurti traveled the world for more than five decades urging us to transform ourselves through self-knowledge and by watching the streams of thoughts and feelings that arise in our minds. He urged his followers to notice the quality of their mental fluctuations and to shift their consciousness to a deeper level of awareness through introspection and reason. Krishnamurti believed this process of self-examination was the key to engendering a fundamental change in society as a whole.

Krishnamurti was born into a Brahmin family, which is the highest caste of Hindu society in India. From an early age, he was seen as an enlightened being by many in India and abroad. The International Theosophical Society, founded in the late 1800s in New York, encouraged the study of comparative religion, philosophy, and science, and was devoted to investigate the unexplained laws of nature and the powers latent in man. Upon meeting Krishnamurti while he was still an adolescent, members of this society were so taken with his presence that they created a worldwide organization, the Order of the Star, to promote him as a guru.

Krishnamurti's Secret to Life

The Theosophical Society brought Krishnamurti to America and established a headquarters in Ojai, California. Krishnamurti soon realized he did not want to be cast as a guru and disavowed the Order of the Star, preferring to teach on his own, urging listeners to explore the basic questions of human existence with honesty, persistence, and open minds. He continued to live in Ojai for several decades, where thousands of admirers would regularly gather to hear him lecture in what is called *satsang*, or 'sitting at the feet of a wise and learned being.' One of Krishnamurti's most memorable teachings was delivered during one of these talks, which I quote from the writings of a student in attendance that day:

'Every spring he (Krishnamurti) used to give talks in a beautiful oak grove... He had been speaking there for over sixty years. On this particular occasion when I went to hear him, in the late 1970s, there must have been close to two thousand people in attendance, sitting on the grass, or in their folding chairs. It was always an extraordinary experience, hearing Krishnamurti in person. Aldous Huxley, who was a friend of Krishnamurti's, described it as: "Like listening to a discourse of the Buddha—such authority, such intrinsic power."

Part way through this particular talk, Krishnamurti suddenly paused, leaned forward, and said, almost conspiratorially, "Do you want to know what my secret is?" Almost as though we were one body, we sat up, even more alert than we had been, if that was possible. I could see people all around me lean forward, their ears straining and their mouths slowly opening in hushed anticipation. Krishnamurti rarely talked about himself or his own process, and now he was about to give us his secret! He was in many ways a mountaintop teacher—somewhat distant, aloof, seemingly unapproachable, unless you were part of his inner circle. Yet that's why we came to Ojai every spring, to see if we could find out just what his secret was. We wanted to know how he managed to be so aware and enlightened, while we struggled with conflict and our numerous problems. There was a silence. Then he said in a soft, almost shy voice, "You see, I don't mind what happens."

I don't mind what happens. This simple statement is the essence of inner freedom. It is a timeless spiritual truth: release attachment to outcomes, and—deep inside yourself—you'll feel good no matter what. You'll feel good because you are connected to, one with, the energy of the universe, the beauty and power of creation itself.' Jim Dreaver

Moving Beyond the Ego

This sounds so simple that I imagine some of the seekers there that day, leaning in to finally hear the great secret of life, were befuddled, confused, or a little disappointed. Many others, like the insightful Jim Dreaver, immediately got the point. What Krishnamurti said that day was a profound teaching, and its practice is potentially life changing. This is because most of us are "minding what happens" all the time. We are deeply attached to outcomes in our lives. We are consumed with our desires and constantly worry that they won't be fulfilled in the way in which we envision. This leads to stress, anxiety, and insecurity.

Beyond this, most of us are caught up in *ahamkara*, the sense that we are the center of the world and it's all about us. This is one of the five *kleshas,* or root causes of suffering as articulated in the Yoga Sutras of Patanjali, which is described as *asmita,* or being overly self-identified (see Chapter Five). We have a vision, which arises from this egocentric point of view, about how our lives should go. We extend this expectation to those around us and to the circumstances that arise in our daily lives. When reality comes along and things turn out differently, we react in various negative ways. We get angry, frustrated, fearful, and depressed. We also become self-absorbed, telling everyone who will listen about our drama and how we have somehow been victimized. Even insignificant matters can trigger this response, and as a result we find ourselves constantly sweating the small stuff. This constant "minding" creates an ongoing state of emotional turmoil.

In shifting to "not minding," we are moving away from the external mind, or *manas*, that controls so much of our awareness, and opening ourselves to understanding reality as it truly is. We then have the opportunity to act in a more intelligent and "mindful" way. This connects us with the aspect of mind called *buddhi*, where our deeper wisdom and intuition dwells.

Krishnamurti's simple little secret is also a teaching of the Bhagavad-Gita. In this profound spiritual text, Krishna is rebuking the warrior Arjuna as he despairs on the battlefield of life. "From the world of the senses, Arjuna, comes heat and comes cold, and pleasure and pain," Krishna teaches. "They come and they go: they are transient. Arise above them strong soul!"

Krishna goes on to remind Arjuna that all of us are embodiments of divine and eternal consciousness. He is implying that we should rise above our individual egos and see the bigger picture.

"The unreal never is," Krishna continues in his conversation with Arjuna, "the real never is not."

This relates to not expecting reality to conform to our egos or our illusions. As Krishna says, "Do thy work in the peace of Yoga and, free from selfish desires, be not moved in success or failure. Yoga is an evenness of mind, a peace that is ever the same." Stop reacting all the time, Krishna is advising, and instead be steady, see things as they are, stand in the peace of Yoga, and do what is required of you in your life.

When we do this, we are no longer "minding what is happening." We are still fully engaged and able to act skillfully instead of reacting and increasing our suffering. Krishna is also advising Arjuna to be detached. This is a central message of the Yoga Sutras of Patanjali as well. The Sutras urge us to have courage, faith, and self-discipline, to practice daily with great intensity, and to remain detached in the process by not seeking a particular outcome. Detachment doesn't mean dropping out of life or sticking our heads in the sand. It means doing the work we need to do for our own personal growth without holding on to preconceived outcomes that arise from the ego. It also means detaching from all the external sensory stimuli in our culture...not buying into the collective illusion of socialization.

From an Ayurvedic standpoint, this detachment and non-reaction also brings great healing. As the mind relaxes, the body relaxes as well. The agitation within us, usually characterized by surges of adrenalin, begins to subside. This sends a signal to our subconscious that we can let down our guard. This relaxed condition is essential to bringing the body back to a state of homeostasis and balance. Further, Ayurveda holds that most of our physical ailments arise from mental imbalances. These imbalances are created by our attachments, aversions, fears, and self-centeredness.

Going with the Flow

You can practice not minding what happens by first coming to see all the ways in which you do react to the circumstances that arise in your daily life. Don't try to change anything at first. Just notice when this happens. You might find you are doing this far more often than you were aware of. Notice how your desires, aversions, or attractions make you internally expect or demand a certain outcome or reality, and try to keep a mental note of these incidents. Notice if you expect those around you to behave in certain ways and if you react when they fail to meet your expectations. Notice, too, what your emotional reactions are even if you are not being demonstrative in any way and are just keeping it inside of you.

It's likely you also will begin to detect that most people around you also are reacting to reality based upon their own personal illusions. Don't judge them for it just because you've started to wake up in this respect, and don't try to teach them the secret. You're likely to cause more reactions within them and run into a wall of resistance. As Krishnamurti taught so often, the primary journey is working on ourselves. This alone can take a lifetime!

Once you become proficient at this process of noticing, begin seeking to make shifts in your perspective. Remind yourself that you are reacting to reality based upon your own illusions. Then, try to let those illusions go. Seek to see the situation for what it really is. Make deliberate choices to ignore the insignificant situations, try go with the flow more often, and then act skillfully when you need to.

Through this process you will gain clarity, insight, and freedom. As you connect with "what is" and openly accept it, you also will be aligning yourself with the higher order of things. You will be moving towards the light. As Krishnamurti himself put it: "When you live with this awareness, this sensitivity, life has an astonishing way of taking care of you. Then there is no problem of security, of what people say or do not say, and that is the beauty of life."

◆ ◆ ◆ ◆ ◆ ◆ ◆ ◆ ◆ ◆

ANCIENT WISDOM
FOR
MODERN TIMES

Your Inner Power

*You have the power
to heal to your maximum potential,
to overcome setbacks
and obstacles,
to find the most authentic you,
live your truth,
and manifest your fullest potential.*

Bhava Ram

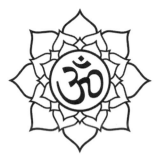

Chapter 11

Pulling the Splinter

Have you ever had a splinter? Isn't it amazing how such a tiny thing can so fully absorb your attention? Everything else seems to lose significance and all you want to do is get that little splinter out. If it's too deep to be extracted with your fingers, or even with tweezers, you might have to use a needle to dig in to get at it or even push the shard out the opposite direction. Ouch. That's how much you want it out. It can be a challenging and painful process, but once the splinter is removed you feel a tremendous sense of relief. Only then can you begin to heal and get on with the more important aspects of your day.

Negative emotions are like splinters. They pierce our consciousness, needle our minds, and consume our thoughts to the point that we feel a constant state of discomfort. Most of us can recall the times we have felt hurt or angered by the harsh words or actions of others, and how we have held on to our pain, processing it over and over in our minds like a never ending one-sided argument. Perhaps we find fear, anger, or stress welling up inside of us as a recurring response to the ups and downs of our daily lives. We often hold onto to these emotional splinters for weeks, months, and even years, so that we become so filled with the piercing slivers of our lives that we wonder if and how we will ever heal from all this pain.

Millions of us end up in therapy, talking for hours with our counselors about these problems we are hanging onto. They put us on antidepressants, leaving us less aware of our worries, but also less aware of life in general. We are still filled with emotional splinters, still irritated, and now we're doped up as well.

The Inner Alchemy of Yoga

Yoga offers a way out, and it doesn't take years of counseling or getting pickled on Prozac. The Yoga Sutras of Patanjali teach us that one powerful practice, called *pratipaksha bhavana*, is a simple yet powerful solution that can be deeply transformative when put into action on a sustained basis.

> **Sutra II.33 *Vitarka Badhane Pratipaksha Bhavanam.***
> "When disturbed by negative thoughts, opposite [positive] ones should be thought of. This is pratipaksha bhavana."

By cultivating an opposite—or positive—thought when we are in the throes of anxiety, we can extract our emotional splinters and pave the way for self-healing. Patanjali is simply asking us to replace anger with compassion, violent thoughts with peaceful ones, hate with love, and even to replace our general feelings of tension and stress with a sense of relaxation and contentment. Holding onto negative thoughts always increases our pain, causing us to be distracted, dysfunctional, and eventually depressed. Such mental illness often leads to physical problems as well and can even lead to serious conditions including heart disease, cancer, stroke, and autoimmune disorders.

Practicing pratipaksha bhavana allows us to release our painful and destructive emotions while creating a new inner chemistry that supports healing and harmony. It involves one of the most important and central principles of Yoga, which is controlling the thought waves of the mind. It also supports several of the Eight Limbs (*Ashtanga*) of Patanjali's Royal (*Raja*) Yoga as articulated in the Sutras. In moving away from external agitation we are practicing the fifth limb, *pratyahara*, which is withdrawing the senses. Through deliberately engaging in a practice of shifting our thoughts, we are practicing the sixth limb of *dharana*, or single-pointed concentration. If we go deeply enough we enter the seventh limb of *dhyana*, or meditation, and ultimately the final limb, *samadhi*, as we become fully absorbed in our practice.

Any of us who have found ourselves in a state of deep anger or hurt know that shifting our feelings is easier said than done. We become psychologically and neurologically habituated to these sharp, dramatic emotions to the point that we often find ourselves over-responding to challenging events, making the tiniest splinter of a perceived negative experience feel like shrapnel piercing our hearts. Over time, this response becomes such an ingrained habit that we often feel unable to control our behavior.

Some of the ways we can practice pratipaksha bhavana during these trying times include simply removing ourselves from a negative situation, leaving the disturbing environment, and finding a place where we can feel safe, peaceful, and calm. We should then try to put the incident into perspective. Is it really the end of the world? Are we overreacting? What might be the consequences of holding onto this? Could we lose a friend, become estranged from a loved one, or just simply ruin our day? Is it really worth all this suffering? How might the outcome be different if we just let it go?

To ease the tension, we can sit for a few minutes and contemplate positive thoughts such as the beauty of nature, the miracle of our breath, or the life of a great sage or saint. We can focus upon cultivating the opposite emotion from the one that has welled up inside of us, such as replacing condemnation with compassion, anger with loving kindness, or fear with courage. We can also choose to see the positive aspects of the person or situation to which we are reacting, or practice self-inquiry (*svadhyaha*) and explore what role we played in creating our drama. If it is a pattern in our lives, we might contemplate how to react differently in the future. This is much more than just counting to ten and letting off the steam, it is teaching ourselves a different way of dealing with life and with our emotions.

In the process we create a new inner chemistry that supports calmness and contentment.

While it is a simple and logical practice, the wisdom of pratipaksha bhavana lies in doing it. If it were a physical splinter, there is no doubt we would take immediate action to pluck it out. Yet all too often we find ourselves holding onto our emotional wounds even when we know we are doing ourselves great harm, resisting the effort to let them go or feeling incapable of doing so. It's as if we lack faith in our capacity to manage our thoughts and emotions, as if they are somehow just happening to us and are beyond our control. While it might often seem this way, Yoga holds that you can take charge. It just takes time and steady practice, which is the key to succeeding at anything in life.

On a deeper level, beyond the obvious self-healing that we can achieve through this practice, pratipaksha bhavana assists us with spiritual transformation and self-realization. The emotions of loving kindness, peace, contentment, and compassion are the natural state of our souls. When we align ourselves with these emotions we move to deeper levels of consciousness and grace. This is best accomplished through deliberate, consistent effort and commitment to ritualized practice.

Pratipaksha Bhavana Practice

Here is one method that I have occasionally taught on retreats and in Deep Yoga classes:

> *Begin seated with your spine tall, your shoulders back, and your heart open. Bring the back of your hands to your knees or thighs, and allow the thumbs and index fingers to touch.*
>
> *Allow whatever negative emotion or experience you wish to deal with to fully arise within your consciousness. Feel the memory of the situation permeate every cell of your being. Really be with it.* One Minute

Release the visualization and let your breath become deep and full, slow and smooth. Balance the breath by silently counting the in-breath and equalizing it with the out-breath. One Minute

Remind yourself of what a privilege it is to be alive. Have gratitude for all the abundance in your life as you feel the grace of each in-breath. Visualize yourself drinking in precious life force from the Universe. See this as a tremendous privilege and blessing. Let each in-breath fill your entire body with light, love and gratitude. Visualize the expansiveness of the cosmos, the smallness of the world, and put your dramas into a broader perspective. Remember that your body is the temple of your spirit, a sacred vessel receiving your breath. One to Two Minutes

Continue the practice as you cultivate a sense that each out-breath is profoundly healing. Release any negative emotions or inner-turbulence down into Mother Earth with every exhale, as you continue contemplating the empowerment, joy and beauty of every inhale. Two to Four Minutes

Now, sit in silence as you notice the inner peace your practice has brought you. Bring your awareness to your heart by crossing your palms over your chest in an embrace of your heart center. Feel love, peace, and contentment radiating from your heart and permeating your entire being. One Minute

With your palms still crossed at the chest, begin the silent mantra of SO HUM (I am that). SO on the in-breath, HUM on the out-breath. Feel yourself as the embodiment of these healing emotions that you have cultivated. One to Two Minutes

Bring your palms together at your heart and chant OM, Shanti, Shanti, Shanti (Peace, Peace, Peace), out loud one time. Bow your head to your heart down towards your heart to seal in the practice.

As you continue your day, try to remember this true nature of your higher self that you have experienced through your practice. Let an occasional in-breath beckon you back to the home of your Soul. Allow an out-breath to be a healing release.

Remember who you truly are and rest in this awareness as you transform your splinters into salve, your anger into compassion, your hate in to love, your fear into courage, your pain into joy. OM, Shanti, Shanti, Shanti (Peace, Peace, Peace).

◆ ◆ ◆ ◆ ◆ ◆ ◆ ◆ ◆ ◆

ANCIENT WISDOM
FOR
MODERN TIMES

Prasadanam

Prasadanam is undisturbed calmness.

*We retain our prasadanam
through cultivating attitudes
of friendliness towards the happy,
delight towards the virtuous,
and disregard for the wicked.*

*Always seek to be in the
company of those who inspire you
to your greatness.*

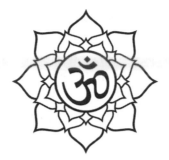

Chapter 12

Wall Street Dharma

Several years ago, when I was battling terminal cancer, a broken back, and a failed back surgery, I abandoned western medicine and fully immersed myself in Yoga as my path to self-healing. There was little time for anything other than seeking to survive, so I simplified my life as much as possible. This included turning my life savings over to an investment advisor. I asked that none of my money be invested in defense, tobacco, or oil stocks, and then forgot the matter, fully devoting myself to *sadhana*, or daily practice of Yoga techniques.

After healing myself and stabilizing my life, I eventually reviewed my portfolio and researched the holdings in the various funds in which I was placed. To my surprise, they included stocks in oil, defense, tobacco, and other corporations completely out of line with my philosophy. I was invested in the very types of activities that Yoga teaches us to avoid as a matter of spiritual principle. How can a practicing Yogi enjoy the full fruits of all that this transformative science has to offer while simultaneously profiting from investments that involve killing, polluting, and plundering? Clearly, I was out of my *dharma,* or right alignment with my beliefs, when it came to Wall Street.

In it's largest sense, dharma is the universal principles of nature, or God's Law if you will. Ayurveda and Yoga seek to align us with these principles in all aspects of our lives. Ayurveda is dharmic medicine. It involves natural healing of the body based upon natural law, and conscious healing of the mind based upon the moral precepts of yogic philosophy. Yoga is dharmic spiritual practice. It involves opening to our higher self and leading our individual lives in accordance with the eternal principles of the universe.

The primary ethic of dharma is the concept of *ahimsa*. Like most Sanskrit words, given the depth and complexity of this ancient language, much is lost in the translation to English. In its most general sense, ahimsa means non-harming or nonviolence. Ahimsa is also one of the Yamas, or principles of social conduct, articulated in the Yoga Sutras of Patanjali that details the eight-limbed path of Yoga.

The practice of ahimsa can be extremely powerful and have widespread effects. Mahatma Gandhi liberated India from oppressive British rule through ahimsa and what he called *satyagraha*, or peaceful noncooperation. Without a single violent act, the most powerful military force in history at the time was forced to retreat and grant India her freedom. This was a key moment in the downfall of Britain's imperialist empire. Martin Luther King, who was deeply influenced by Gandhi, led the American Civil Rights Movement through satyagraha and achieved remarkable progress for equality and social evolution.

The dharma of peace and harmony is what we seek to achieve through all our Yoga practices, from our pranayama breath work, asana postures, mantras, and meditations, to the alignment of our lifestyles. This, of course, includes not committing any sort of violence against our fellow brothers and sisters on the planet. It also involves embracing all peoples, all ethnicities, religions, societies, and countries as part of the beautiful and multicolored fabric of humankind.

So essential is peace to the health of the individual body and mind, to our communities, our nations, and to the very health of the planet, that we are asked through Yoga to support peace in every possible way, starting with ensuring that our lives are founded on ahimsa.

In conducting recent wars in the Middle East, the United States has poured hundreds of billions of dollars into the coffers of defense contractors. Knowing this, many mutual fund managers have moved large portions of their portfolios into companies sure to profit from these conflicts. This includes non-defense corporations as well, such as multinational oil companies that are reporting billions of dollars in record profits as a direct result of the higher oil prices created by the wars.

During the run-up to these wars, corporations involved in our military/industrial complex lobbied their Senators and members of Congress extensively for the lucrative contracts they knew would soon be available. This led to reports of corruption and bribery, and the indictment and conviction of several lobbyists and politicians who were most blatant in their conduct. We also have seen hundreds of millions of dollars lost to fraud and waste in these contracts. This constitutes a form of violence against the democratic principles of our nation.

Tobacco companies are often a favorite of investment advisors for their high dividends and stable profits. While these corporations are not involved in war, they are involved in violence through the deaths that result from tobacco related diseases. This includes tens of thousands of Americans ever year who die of lung cancer from smoking. Tobacco companies practice a more subtle form of violence with their advertising campaigns that often target our youth in hopes of creating addiction early on. The have a history of false claims about the benefits of tobacco and continuously seek to deny or obfuscate the dangers of smoking.

When I realized that my investments were out of line with dharma, I immediately liquidated the account. With a little research on the Internet, I found several socially responsible investment funds, called SRI's, that screen out any investments in defense, oil, tobacco, alcohol, animal testing, environmental damage, or Third World exploitation. The financial performance of these funds is typically lower than the funds investing in war and exploitation, but I believe it is a price well worth paying.

Food as a Gesture of Peace

The practice of ahimsa goes far beyond war and human conflict. It also includes cultivating a mental attitude of wishing no injury to any part of the natural order of life. This is a primary reason that Yoga and Ayurveda recommend a vegetarian diet. As my Ayurvedic teacher, Dr. David Frawley puts it, "Food should not be based on cruelty. Food, after all, is a means of providing nourishment. What kind of nourishment can be derived from food that reflects not the energy of love but that of exploitation?"

While I do not advocate a pure vegetarian diet in all circumstances, we humans are designed to be herbivores, not carnivores, and our overconsumption of meat, which is often tainted with preservatives, antibiotics, and hormones, is at the root of many of the major health problems facing our nation today. A variety of studies have shown that the three major killers—cancer, heart attack, and stroke—are significantly lower among those who eat vegetarian diets.

When we buy and consume meat produced by factory farms we are not only ingesting the poisons they put into the animals to boost their profits, we are helping to sustain the violence they commit against these animals by keeping them crowded together in torturous conditions. If we do choose to eat animals, humanely raised, free range and wild caught products are the optimal choice both for health reasons and for the practice of ahimsa.

Ahimsa has more subtle aspects as well. It includes not engaging in personal actions that are destructive, manipulative, deceptive, or exploitative. If we ridicule, manipulate, or dominate those around us we are engaging in psychological violence. If we gossip or spread negative stories about others it is also a subtle form of harming. If we use profanity or harsh speech we are out of alignment with the dharma of ahimsa. If we obtain and horde too many possessions, which is common in our culture these days, it can also be a form of harming the environment through the over-harvesting of natural resources to create nonessential consumer goods. If the goods we buy come from the exploited labor of Third World countries, we are engaging in an even subtler form of harming.

As you can see already, there is a great deal involved with this one simple word: Ahimsa. The dharma of Ayurveda and Yoga asks a great deal of us. To align ourselves with the universal principles of nature we must have determination, discipline, and commitment. The result of this challenging work is a life more in harmony with ourselves and our world, greater physical and emotional well being, and—most importantly—a spiritual wellness that brings us the contentment and inner peace that no external possessions, no power, no wealth, and no high-performing mutual fund can ever provide.

A Life of Non-Harming

Yoga invites us to contemplate ahimsa on a daily basis and, what is more important, to practice integrating it into our lives. As a beginning, I invite you to review your life and make a list of ways in which you might cause less harm. It might be as simple as committing to recycling or consuming less. You also might find ways in which you have been causing harm that you were completely unaware of, and perhaps you will decide it's time to make a change. As you grow your awareness and commitment to ahimsa, you will move more deeply into dharma and therein find a rich and subtle peace in life.

◆ ◆ ◆ ◆ ◆ ◆ ◆ ◆ ◆ ◆

ANCIENT WISDOM
FOR
MODERN TIMES

Guru

*In Sanskrit,
gu means darkness,
ru is light.*

*The gurus is the
one who helps us to move
from the darkness
to the light.*

*The greatest guru you will know
is you.*

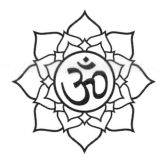

Chapter 13
Breath of Life

There once were three kings who ruled the entire world. Their kingdoms had grown to span the globe and, inevitably, their borders began to butt up against one another. This eventually caused disputes, suspicion and enmity to break out between them. All attempts at diplomacy and compromise failed. Finally, the kings found themselves on the brink of a great conflict. Mighty armies were amassed on the borders of their empires and the stage was set for a veritable holocaust.

On the eve of this impending disaster, a Great Spirit descended from the heavens and brought the three kings before her on the battlefield. "Tomorrow, you will do great harm to the whole world if you wage this war," she admonished them, "so I have decided to give each of you a single boon. This way one of you, the one who makes the wisest choice, will immediately prevail and much bloodshed will be avoided."

The Spirit explained that everything else would be taken away from each king—everything—and, come the morning, each would have only his one boon upon which to rely. She then announced that she would see each of them individually to learn of their choice so that the others wouldn't know what decision their adversaries had made.

When his turn for a private audience came, the first king, who was deeply attached to power, quickly told the Spirit that the boon he chose was to be given all the soldiers and weapons on earth. This way, he cleverly thought, the other kings would be defenseless. He would quickly vanquish them, their armies would surrender, and he alone would rule the world.

The Spirit smiled, and said, "So be it."

The second king, whose great passion was for wealth, was just as fast with his decision, asking the Spirit for all the gold, silver, gems, and treasure in the world. Also thinking himself very clever, he figured he would spend the night bribing all the supporters of the other two kings, promising them the riches his boon would deliver in the morning, and then he would quickly vanquish his adversaries.

The Spirit smiled, and said, "So be it."

The third king, who alone had unsuccessfully sought peace with the others and felt no desire for conflict, came before the Spirit humbly and without hurry. He bowed at her feet and asked for forgiveness for whatever role he had played in creating this mess.

"Oh Great Spirit," he said reverently, "at first, for my boon, I thought of asking that you be on my side. There is no doubt that, with your might, all my foes immediately would be overcome. However, I have no desire for this battle and do not wish to see all the suffering, death, and destruction that will surely result from such a terrible war. So I ask for this: take all that I have, only leave me the gift of my breath. I will gladly give up everything else in hopes of ending this enmity."

The Spirit smiled, and said, "So be it."

When dawn arrived, The Spirit gathered the three kings again on the battlefield and granted their boons. The first king immediately was surrounded by all the soldiers and weapons on earth, but soon began gasping for his breath and quickly realized that no army could save his life. The second king saw all the world's wealth pile up behind him, but he, too, began gulping for air and immediately realized that all the riches on earth were not enough not purchase his life. In their final moments of life, both kings gazed at the third king, who was breathing easily, and realized that he alone had made the correct decision. With their final gasps, they surrendered their boons of power and wealth to the surviving king, ordering their people to unite behind him as their sovereign ruler.

The Miracle of Breath

Of the many gifts you have in your life, there is none so sacred and essential as your breath. The first thing you do when you enter this world is to take a breath. The last thing you do when you depart this world is to take a breath. In the most tangible of ways, breath IS life. The most ancient, time-tested, effective way to begin and sustain the journey of self-realization is through the miracle of your breath. The easiest way to reduce stress is through the miracle of your breath. A key to detoxifying your body is through the miracle of your breath. A quick passageway into the present moment is through the miracle of your breath.

If you were in some kind of crisis, say a war or natural disaster, you might be amazed at your ability to survive incredible hardship and deprivation. Of course, some of us would cope better than others based upon our strength, health, outlook, and constitution. Still, most of us could go for days without water. We could survive even longer without food. We have the capacity to endure a lack of light, human contact, warmth, or shelter for far longer than most of us realize. But none of us would live more than five minutes under any circumstances without our breath.

Your breath is the most essential, powerful, and precious aspect of your physical existence. It's worth more than all the fortune and fame in the world and yet, amazingly when you think about it, it's absolutely free—a gift of life from the Divine. It's a gift that most of us take for granted and most of us underutilize. The average person breathes at only about one-third of their capacity, and this shallowness of respiration is the source of much physical and emotional discomfort.

The Science of Breath

There are some seventy-five to one hundred trillion cells in the human body. Each cell is designed to be like an individual energy factory; pulsating, vibrating and "breathing" as it transforms oxygen and food into biological energy. Scientists have labeled each minuscule speck of this energy as adenosine triphosphate, or ATP, and refer to it as 'the currency of life.' Without ATP, there is no energy and therefore no life. Plants create it through photosynthesis. Animals produce ATP primarily through respiration and secondarily through breaking down the energy in food. ATP literally permeates all living matter and dwells at the core, cellular level of every living thing.

Every time you blink an eye, flex a muscle, "fire" a brain cell, fight a cold, or make an effort to do anything, you are accessing the energy of ATP. To determine how much ATP you make and use every day just weigh yourself. If you are, say, 150 pounds and reasonably healthy and active, you are making and burning 150 pounds of ATP every day. So, logically, the more ATP you create the more energy and power you possess. The more your inner power, the better you feel, the more quickly you heal, the more you are able to live a vibrant, healthy, and productive life. When your ATP production is low or interrupted, you experience "energy outages" that can result in symptoms from mild fatigue to life-threatening illness. While you might want to eat the most energy rich, purest food possible, you cannot stuff yourself to the gills in hopes of boosting your ATP.

You can, however, significantly increase your ATP through your breath. Yet most of us take the miracle of our breath for granted and rely on our autonomic nervous system to do the breathing for us. As a result, we create less ATP, contain less energy, and "burn less brightly" than our full potential. It's little wonder so many of us feel like our lives are ordinary, mundane, and less fulfilling than we would like. While there are a host of other factors that contribute to our emotional states and our perspectives on the world, at the very core of our ability to perform and to experience the fullness of our lives is the potency of our life force, or level of ATP.

Yoga and the Science of Breath

Yogis have focused on the power of the breath for thousands of years. What modern day science calls ATP is known as *prana* in Sanskrit. The pranic energy in each cell of our bodies is seen as a reflection of the light and the power of the sun, which is considered the source of all energy, and from a yogic perspective is central to our connection with the Universe. Scientists have now concluded that our solar system and the planets were formed following the explosion of stars into supernovas. The space between our sun and the Earth is filled with tiny, energized particles of "star stuff" called plasma. This plasma is the lifeblood of the Universe and the most common form of matter. We arise from this, and therefore we truly are stardust. ATP can be called our own inner-stardust...cosmic energy itself.

Pranayama is the Yogic science of increasing ATP in our cells and throughout our bodies as a whole. Through deep and regulated breathing, we not only increase our life force, we reduce stress, release negative emotions, diminish physical pain, and promote both psychological and physiological healing, balance, and wellness. Pranayama, therefore, is a primary form of yogic medicine and central to self-healing.

Newcomers to Yoga often find it easy to connect with the transformative power of postures, or asanas, because they can feel the stretch in their hamstrings and lower back, the opening in their hips, or the challenge of a balance pose. Connecting with the breath through the practice of pranayama is more elusive because it's much subtler. It takes time to begin the process of stilling the mind, moving away from external stimuli, and entering deeper states of awareness. Yogic texts even warn beginners to always practice pranayama under the guidance of a seasoned teacher since it can disturb and agitate the unprepared.

While pranayama is subtler than asana, it's much more powerful. While this is challenging for novices and even many devoted practitioners to comprehend, it becomes clear with dedicated practice over a sustained period of time. Awareness of the breath also has a transformative and spiritual component. Connecting with our breath brings us into the inner practices of Patanjali's *Ashtanga*, or Eight Limbs of Yoga. It promotes the final three limbs: Pratyahara (withdrawal of the senses), Dharana (single-pointed concentration), and Dhyana (meditation). Many meditative practices are based upon mastering the breath or merely "watching the breath" in silence and stillness. Breathing is an exchange between our inner world and the outer world. It is a flow of the masculine and feminine, receiving and giving, a dance of body, mind, and Spirit as one. It is, in essence, a perpetual celebration of life.

While we should seek instruction and guidance with technical pranayama techniques, we can experience both the healing and transformative qualities offered by the breath simply through teaching ourselves to breathe more deeply throughout our daily lives. We don't need a Yoga studio to practice this, nor an instructor or special time set aside. We can do it most anywhere we like. All we need is to increase our attention and make a minimal effort on a sustained basis.

Daily Breath of Life

You might want to start by remembering how sacred the breath is when you wake up in the morning. Let this be your cue to begin breathing deeply and fully, always through the nose when possible as it is our natural organ of the breath and acts as a filter of the air. Teach yourself to breathe in a three-part Yogic breath, filling first your belly, then your ribs, then your chest. Exhale chest, ribs, belly. To deepen this technique, let your abdomen inflate like a potbelly on the inhalation. At the bottom of the exhalation, contract your abdominal muscles and draw your navel towards the spine.

Seek to practice these deep and full breaths throughout your day. You can do this at your desk, standing in a grocery line, driving your car, or taking a walk. Of course, you will often forget your breath and revert to automatic pilot. Every time you notice this, recall the sacredness of the breath and return to deep breathing.

In time, you will create a new, deeper and fuller pattern of breathing. You may begin to notice that you have more energy, greater balance, and less stress in your life. Once the pattern is established, it's time to contemplate more deeply how the breath connects you to the Divine. Slowly allow yourself to open to the fullness and the grace of your existence as expressed through the sacredness of your precious breath. This awareness alone will guide you deeper into the interior spaces of your being. In the process, you will build your ATP from a scientific perspective and build your inner light from a Yogic point of view, as the Spirit of Breath literally moves you towards en*light*enment.

◆ ◆ ◆ ◆ ◆ ◆ ◆ ◆ ◆ ◆

ANCIENT WISDOM
FOR
MODERN TIMES

Tapas

Tapas is self-disciple.

It is stoking the inner fire
of transformation.

Tapas is the essence
of courage, faith, and focus.

Tapas is the key to success
in all that you aspire to.

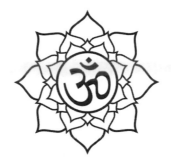

Chapter 14

Yoga of the Heart

You may have been asked at some point in a Yoga class to "open your heart," either through mental intention or the physical motion of drawing your shoulders back and bringing your chest forward, or by entering into a backbend. For some of us the idea of opening our hearts can seem a bit strange or hard to grasp. We know a backbend gives us a challenging stretch and opens the spine, but what does this have to do with "opening our hearts" during our practice? Is there such a thing as a heart-opening pose or attitude, or is this just flowery Yoga rap intended to sound deep and spiritual?

We can explore this in several ways. In this essay I've chosen to focus on the Chakras. Chakra is a Sanskrit word that means wheel or vortex. Most Yogic texts articulate seven primary chakras in the body, running from the area of the tailbone up to the crown of the head. The New Age movement has latched onto chakras and marketed all sorts of chakra kits with colored stones, charts, and creative drawings that frankly trivialize the science behind these vital energy centers. There is much more to them, not only in a spiritual sense, but in a physiological context as well.

Each of the seven chakras is associated with one of the seven endocrine glands and with a group of nerves called a plexus. While the chakras are very subtle and cannot be removed or dissected like body parts, these energy vortices function like invisible power plants of our energy system and consciousness. Our chakras open, close, and swirl as we think, feel, respond, and react to the world around us. This is analogous to those times in our lives when we have a "gut feeling," a "lump in our throat," or "feeling in our heart" about a significant or challenging event in our lives. Chakras hold much of the instinct and intelligence passed down to us through our DNA. They also contain memory, which plays a significant role in triggering our habituated responses to life.

When we are born we function through the root chakra, called *muladhara*, located near the base of the tailbone. This is where the primal "fight or flight" response is generated and is associated with survival. After a few years, we gain consciousness in the second chakra, *swadhisthana*, located between the pubis and navel. Here we begin to interact with the world around us, explore desires and grab things within our reach, yet still perceive everything as a part of us and not separate. By age seven or eight we open at chakra three, *manipura*, located in the region of the navel. Here we begin to establish our individuality. This chakra governs ego, our level of self-centeredness, our desire for power, possessions, control, self-assertion, and taking charge of our own lives.

While the first three chakras are more complex than the simple overview offered here and have many more functions and aspects, I mention the qualities above because this is where many of us dwell throughout our lives. When we get stuck in the lower chakras, they often become deficient or imbalanced in a manner that leaves us living on the edge of fear and anger without even knowing it. This makes us centered upon ourselves, acting from the ego, seeking possessions, material pleasures, power, and control. When challenge and crisis arise, we instinctively react through these first three chakras, and often these reactions only serve to make matters worse.

Strong lower chakra emotions of ego, selfishness, anger, and fear all create specific neurochemicals that course through our bodies each time they are triggered. This can happen in very simple every day experiences, like when a speeding driver cuts you off on the freeway and you instantly feel road rage. A common modern malady associated with this fight or flight phenomenon is adrenal fatigue. It often goes like this:

- The stress and fast pace of our lives causes mental agitation.
- The lower chakras activate and our adrenal glands pump out adrenalin.
- The sympathetic nervous system is on high alert and cannot relax.
- We can't seem to control our negative emotional habit patterns no matter how clearly we understand that they are doing us harm.
- This, in turn, increases our tension and agitation.

This cycle of emotional toxicity is like self-poisoning ourselves, and it eventually leads to psychological and physiological diseases. This is where opening our hearts comes in. The fourth chakra, *anahata*, is located in the spiritual heart-center right behind the breastbone and is associated, of course, with the organ of the heart. Anahata chakra is our energy center of compassion, gratitude, acceptance, peace, and loving kindness. It is also, according to Yoga and Ayurveda, our true seat of consciousness and the origin of the mind.

I have a son who is one of the most loving, kind, and easygoing people that I have ever known. Yet there have been times when I have found myself close to losing patience and going into a "lower chakra" reaction over something that I soon come to realize is trivial in the larger scheme of life. When I feel this way, I stop myself and place my hand over my heart and whisper, "I love you, everything is okay." He always places his hand over his heart and answers, "I love you too, daddy." As we both think and feel from our hearts, whatever felt stressful between us is quickly diffused, and the bond between us grows even deeper.

This idea of thinking with the heart can be a challenging concept, especially since western science has traditionally held the view that the mind is completely contained in the brain. Mass media, which permeates our lives, assaults our brains with fast-paced images and scenarios that accelerate the pace of our externalized minds. As a result, we find ourselves "in our heads" most of the time, cut off from the heart and from the deeper wisdom and serenity it contains.

Western science is now just beginning to catch up with the science of Yoga. Researchers have determined that sixty percent of heart cells are neural cells, which function similarly to those in the brain, thus confirming the heart truly is an organ of perception. This is worth repeating: Your heart is an organ of perception. Further, your heart is capable of producing a magnetic energy field that is five thousand times stronger than the energy field of your brain. This "heart field" can be detected up to ten feet away by sensitive scientific instruments. According to Yoga, this field is the energy of love, and the more we develop it the greater our compassion, inner peace, and awareness.

The Power of Offering the Heart

Mahatma Gandhi, the great Yogi who led India to independence from British rule, performed a stunning political and social "miracle of the heart" in 1947 as the transition to his country's independence was underway. In the city of Calcutta, traditional animosity between Muslims and Hindus had boiled over into rage and violence. Marauding gangs from both sides had been clashing for months. Tens of thousands were wounded and more than four thousand people were killed, many of them innocent women, children, and elderly. In the midst of this chaos, at age 78, Gandhi traveled to Calcutta and announced he would fast until the violence ceased or his life ended. Within five days, Gandhi achieved what no military force could. He opened the hearts of warring Hindus and Muslims alike, moving them into a realm of higher consciousness through his love and his willingness to sacrifice his life. In effect, he became the heart of every citizen in Calcutta as he miraculously transformed the violence into peace.

Yoga of the Heart

So, to answer my own rhetorical question at the beginning of this chapter, heart openings in our practice are very real and can have a profound affect upon our lives. Traditional Hatha Yoga is an energetic practice with many asanas, such as backbends for the heart, designed to energize the chakras and move pranic energy up the spine. This practice helps us to move past the lower chakras and into higher levels of awareness. Energy is a form of light, and moving this energy upwards is why we call the result of spiritual practice en*light*enment.

The final three chakras above the heart, *vishuddhi*, *ajna*, and *sahashara*, respectively at the throat, eyebrow center, and crown of the head, hold more advanced aspects of consciousness that are accessed through devoted practice over a long period of time. For most of us, however, it is accomplishment enough to open our hearts.

Two of the greatest texts of Yoga, the Yoga Sutras of Patanjali and the Bhagavad-Gita, both guide us towards the heart center as a primary place upon which to meditate. When we open our hearts through postures, mental intention, and meditation, we not only connect with our true nature of love and bliss; we also enter into a deeper dialogue with the inner wisdom of our Spirit. This is essential for leaving behind habituated and unconscious responses to life. It is a pathway to self-healing, personal growth, and transformation. Viewing life from the heart allows us to become more open and accepting of reality, less controlling or frustrated when things don't go the way we had planned, and less reactive and emotional when the inevitable challenge or crisis arises.

An Open Heart Practice

As an experiment, try focusing on your heart during Asana practice, even if you are not prompted to do so by your teacher. Think, feel, and experience Yoga from the "mind in your heart." Notice the energy of your heart chakra opening and expanding in backbends. Breathe golden light into your heart center, then hold your breath for a few seconds and allow it to permeate every cell of your being. Have the intention of moving from the lower chakras to the eternal flame of love, peace, compassion, gratitude, acceptance, and—perhaps most importantly—true self-acceptance and inner wisdom of your heart. When you bring your palms together in *anjali mudra* (prayer mudra) at the close of your practice, remind yourself that saying *namaste* is an act of bowing from the glowing light in your heart to the light in the hearts of your teacher and fellow Yogis in your class. It is also a recognition of the light that glows in the hearts of all humankind and animates all life on Mother Earth, reminding us that we are all truly one.

Try taking this experience up from your Yoga mat and bringing it in your daily life where we all need it most. Inevitably, stressful stuff will happen, and your lower chakras will fire up and get you ready to fight. When this occurs, begin by bringing your palms together at your chest as a reminder of heart consciousness. Then see your body as the temple of your Spirit. Visualize the radiant light of love that glows within your heart. Unfold this field of light and see it expand around you, embracing the situation and everyone and everything involved in it. From this place of awareness, allow the wisdom of your heart to prevail, and watch as the situation seems to resolve itself in far better fashion than you ever expected. Then, silently, whisper "namaste" to yourself and give thanks to the glowing light of the conscious mind within your beautiful and sacred heart.

◆ ◆ ◆ ◆ ◆ ◆ ◆ ◆ ◆ ◆

ANCIENT WISDOM
FOR
MODERN TIMES

Samskara

*Samaskaras are deep-seated
impressions in our subconscious
that create habits
that are often difficult to overcome.*

*The practices of Yoga
assist us in overcoming samskaras
and therein transform our lives.*

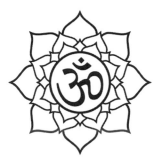

Chapter 15
Rainbow Waterfall

High up a beautiful mountainside, nestled against a thick forest, sat an ancient village. It was perfectly situated and stayed cool and pleasant when the summer heat baked the valley below. In winter, the tall trees provided a bulwark from passing storms. Everyone had meaningful work and food was abundant. Yet, despite having all this in their favor, the people were deeply unhappy. There was widespread bitterness, division, and anger amongst them. Arguments broke out daily within families and between families, at the workplace, and at home. Others simply spent their days in anxiety, apprehension, sadness and fear.

The villagers were convinced that their troubles stemmed from a great boulder that had fallen from a peak long ago, landing smack in the middle of the only path up the mountainside. Legend held that somewhere high above that boulder was a magical Rainbow Waterfall. Their folklore told them that all who drank from its waters found a deep sense of peace and tranquility. Their ancestors had lived in such a state of happiness and harmony, back before the boulder broke away from the mountain above and blocked the trail. With no access to the Rainbow Waterfall, the villagers now felt lost and alone.

One day a wandering sage arrived in the village. This hadn't happened in more than a century, and the people soon gathered round him.

"You are a wise man sent to help us," one woman said, "please come move the great boulder from the mountain trail so we can get to our Rainbow Waterfall!"

"Yes," the others chimed in, "we are miserable and you must help us!"

"I'll see what can be done," said the sage as he walked through the village with all the townspeople in tow, finding his way up the narrow path to the great boulder.

Upon arriving, the sage gazed up, scratched his chin and calmly said, "Yes, it surely is a big stone."

"We've tried everything," the villagers responded, "from roping it and pulling it with our strongest teams of oxen to cutting down mighty trees and trying to pry it loose. It's impossible to move!"

"Yes, Yes, okay," the sage softly replied, "but, you see, there's no need to move it."

"What do you mean?" several people cried out, beginning to feel anger at this small and gentle man. "Are you a fake? Are you powerless to help us?"

"You can just go around it," he said softly, as he pointed to a steep incline, "just climb that cliff beside the boulder and you'll find your Rainbow Waterfall."

Well, that didn't sit too well with anyone. There were many strict rules in the village, all designed to keep order, and one paramount rule was that people should stay on the narrow paths leading into and out of the village and not stray into unknown territory. Besides, the villagers pointed out, look at how steep and craggy the rocky cliffs were on both sides of the boulder—which was quite true—and how impossibly foolish, dangerous, and difficult it would be to attempt such an ascent!

"Sometimes you have to make the greatest of efforts," the sage told them encouragingly, "and if you do, you'll find that you can do that which you felt you were incapable of doing. Just watch me. I'm an old man, and if I can get up there safely, so can you."

With that, the sage slipped off his sandals and scampered barefoot up the towering rocks as nimbly as could be. Within minutes, he was out of sight. The amazed villagers began to murmur; some calling out that the old sage would surely never make it down again. To their surprise, he was soon climbing deftly back down, with a wet, glistening beard and a big smile on his face.

"It's a beautiful waterfall," he said, chuckling with glee, "and its water tastes like nectar!"

A village elder pushed through the crowd and stepped forth, confronting the sage.

"This is wrong," he cried out, "in our village we never stray off the narrow path in anything we do. That would be against our rules! We must stick to our ways! Anyway, we could never make that climb. You must have created some sort of mystical illusion!"

There were cries of agreement, clenched fists, and folded arms. The old sage could see and feel their resistance and it made him sigh deeply.

"As you wish," he said sadly, "I'll be going now."

And with that, he began to clamber up the other side of the boulder, which was even steeper, and soon vanished into the thin mountain air.

The villagers were crestfallen as the elder ordered them back to their homes. But, the following morning, a few brave souls gathered before sunrise and quietly slipped out of town and up the narrow path to the great boulder. Helping and encouraging one another, they began climbing the steep cliff into which it was wedged, trying to follow the route the old sage had taken. To their dismay, it was extremely difficult, they slipped and fell and scraped their skin and found themselves even more amazed at how easy the old sage had made it look.

After an hour or so, with some torn fingernails and plenty of bruises, they gave up for the day, yet they vowed to meet again the following morning and stay at it every day until they succeeded. As the weeks turned into months, some lost their courage and dropped out, declaring it was impossible, and reminding the others that it also was against the rules. The others, however, stayed with it despite their setbacks and frustrations. Each day they became a little stronger and more flexible, their focus increased, and their commitment deepened.

Finally, after many months, the first of them made it to the top. Just as their lore had promised—and the old sage had confirmed—they came back down refreshed, peaceful, and happy from journey. The rest of the group eventually made it as well, and they, too, were transformed. They found they were no longer bothered by all the troubles plaguing their village. They were happier, healthier, less argumentative, and more relaxed. No matter what happened around them, they were at peace.

Other villagers quietly began to join them, inspired by their example, and eventually accepted them as teachers and guides who could show them they way to the Rainbow Waterfall. In time, almost everyone made the ascent to the sacred waters. Those who had pioneered the way became the new village elders, and they all lived happily ever after.

Making a Shift

The villagers who sneaked up that narrow path that following morning after the sage departed had *intention*. They had made a *shift* away from the status quo of their lives and towards personal growth. They tapped into their *inner power*, released old agreements about their capacity to chart the course of their lives, and finally, most importantly, they committed to *sustained effort*.

Some also dropped out. It's never easy to scale to new heights with the weight of our old ways pulling us down like gravity. This is why all the positive thought, intention setting, visualization, and imagining in the world can only take us so far. To get over the top, to reach the Rainbow Waterfall, we have to *commit ourselves to taking action...to* making a real effort over time.

Reggae star Jimmy Cliff made it into a memorable song:

You can get it if you really want
You can get it if you really want
You can get it if you really want,
But you must try, try and try
Try and try, you'll succeed at last.

Okay. Most of us have heard this from parents all of our lives. So what's new? Remember the difference between knowledge and wisdom. Knowledge is information. Wisdom is putting the information into action...it's doing rather than just knowing and understanding. This is the true secret. You have to know what you want. You have to really want it. Then, you have to try and try, try and try. Stick with it, you WILL succeed at last!

A final note on the Rainbow Waterfall: When the villagers stepped off the narrow path and made the climb around the great boulder, there was a stream with a small waterfall, but except for the reflection created by the sun glancing through the cascading water, there was no rainbow...no magic elixir.

What transformed the villagers was the journey itself, the process of stepping into unknown territory, sustaining their ascension with great effort, and reaching their goal. The magic elixir was finding their inner power, with which they connected through the act of taking charge of their lives, believing in themselves, letting go of old agreements, stepping outside the boundaries, and making a shift. It worked. It always does!

Climbing to the Rainbow Waterfall

All quick fixes are false promises. To make the shifts we need to enhance our lives we must make a sustained effort. There are no exceptions to this eternal law. None.

You have the power of transformation inside of you, no matter how many times you have tried and failed, you have it. The key is to start small, go slowly, a little bit at a time. If we take on too much, try to reach enlightenment overnight, we are just creating more doing in our lives and setting ourselves up for failure.

Choose something small and easily doable. Do you want to exercise? Be in nature more often? Cut down on unnecessary activities? Find more stillness and silence? Take a moment and go through the Eight Steps Into Yoga (see appendix). In that relaxed state, ask your heart, *'Where should I begin?'* You'll get the right answer. Trust it. Then embrace it.

Make a plan now. Climb towards your chosen Rainbow Waterfall for a few minutes every day. Just a few minutes. You can find the time by simply cutting back on those activities that are merely distractions, shortening your to-do list, clicking off the tube.

Stay with it no matter what. There will be slips and falls, torn nails and bruises as you climb. Expect them. Embrace them. Thank them. Don't ever forget that you CAN get it, if you REALLY want it. Don't worry about the outcome. Don't get anxious for the result. Just stay with it. Try and try, gently, try and try. Before you know it, and usually when you least expect it, you will realize you are there. Your Rainbow Waterfall will be right there in front of you. Drink its nectar, splash it on your face...dive in and make a cannonball!

◆ ◆ ◆ ◆ ◆ ◆ ◆ ◆ ◆ ◆ ◆

ANCIENT WISDOM
FOR
MODERN TIMES

From the Upanishads

As your desire is,
so is your will.

As your will is,
so is your deed.

As your deed is,
so is your destiny.

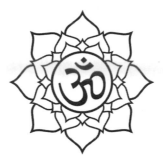

Chapter 16
Gratitude

Your life seems filled with stress, there is never enough time to complete your task list, work is dreadful, relationships are a challenge, and you find yourself anxious, fearful, angry, and dissatisfied.

Has this ever happened to you? Then you get a wicked cold. As it hits you with its full force, you look back to those terrible times you were experiencing just days earlier and they don't seem so bad anymore. All you want now is for the cold to go away. Just feeling normal would be a blessing—even with all the frustrations that seemed so overwhelming just a short time before.

Singer/songwriter Joni Mitchell memorialized this shifting emotional process decades ago, in 1970, with the hit song "Big Yellow Taxi." She bemoaned the destruction of nature, paradise being paved over for parking lots, and the loss of relationship. The essence of her insight was embodied in the verse "don't it always seem to go that you don't know what you've got till it's gone?" This is such a profound and pervasive truth that the taxi song has been recorded by artists throughout the years and has been used in several movie soundtracks.

Don't It Always Seem To Go?

All too often, we take the true blessings in our lives for granted, as if they were our birthright, and we fixate on the things that irritate us. In the process, we miss out on much of the joy of daily life, unaware that our aggravation is a choice, and that it arises from illusion.

"What do you mean?" some might exclaim indignantly, "My overbearing, controlling, belittling, deceitful boss is not my choice nor an illusion!"

This might be true enough, but your *reaction* to the situation *is* your choice. You can choose to loathe this person with authority over you, complain to your colleagues, let it gnaw away at you, and cultivate profound self-pity over your plight. The result of this choice will be an increased level of stress, unhappiness, and lack of vocational fulfillment. It won't, however, change the behavior of your boss in the slightest.

Instead of creating a personal drama like this, you can choose instead to assess the situation and use it for personal advancement. You can explore what part of your negative feelings might be a projection of your own personality issues. You can seek options, such as entering into dialogue with your boss in hopes of finding common ground. You can determine to find a new job in a fashion that doesn't threaten your economic security or career goals. Or you can choose to focus on the aspects of your work that you find rewarding rather than fixate on your frustrations. The key is to not react to the situation or create drama, but to see it for what it truly is and take skillful action.

Overcoming Illusions

This is where ending our illusions enters the equation. The world is never what our ego and self-centeredness demands that it be. Not everyone will see the greatness we see in ourselves or constantly seek to affirm us. The sun won't shine warmly every time we have a picnic. We plan, God laughs. Life is what happens, not what we expect or often demand that it be. This expectation and demand is our illusion. Our reactions to situations that don't fit our illusion are at the root of our suffering. For instance, if you were fired from that miserable job, you might unconsciously shift perspectives and begin to mourn your loss, suddenly realizing how fond you were of your colleagues, how rewarding much of the work was, and you might even recall times when your boss gave you praise. Again, by choice, you would be suffering. *Don't it always seem to go...?*

Your choice of reactions to life has only increased your pain. You might also notice that much of the negative self-talk in your mind is based upon reactions to a reality that fails to conform to your illusory expectations. It's likely that you are not seeing the full reality, but instead viewing it through the constricted prism of your smaller self, or ego. This, again, is "being in the kleshas" as discussed earlier, and a prominent cause of our suffering.

Making a Shift

Yoga advises us repeatedly to break out of this cycle. In the Bhagavad-Gita, Krishna lectures the mighty warrior, Arjuna, as he faces his dark side on the great battlefield of life, telling him that he must see life as it is, be free from selfish desire, unmoved by failure or success, and abide ever in an even and peaceful state of mind.

Verses II:62-65 provide a powerful summary of Krishna's message:

"When a person dwells on the pleasures of sense, attraction for them arises in them. From attraction arises desire, the lust of possession, and this leads to passion, to anger. From passion comes confusion of mind, then loss of remembrance, then forgetting of duty. From this loss comes the ruin of reason, and the ruin of reason leads to destruction. But the soul that moves in the world of senses and yet keeps the senses in harmony, free from attractions and aversions, finds rest in quietness. In this quietness falls down the burden of all sorrows, for when the heart has found quietness, wisdom also has found peace."

The Yoga Sutras of Patanjali, provides a host of practices to still the fluctuations of our minds, cultivate steadiness and calmness, and remain undisturbed by the shifting circumstances of our lives. The Sutras advise us to arise above our petty concerns and desires and place our awareness at the highest level. Patanjali outlines this in the Niyamas, or personal observances of practice, which we might also call our relationship with ourselves:

Sutra II:32 *Sauca samtosa tapah svadhyay yesvera pranidhanani niyamah.*

Niyama consists of purity, contentment, self-discipline, spiritual studies, and a constant awareness of God.

Patanjali suggests that we should see God—or Ishvara in Sanskrit—within ourselves and within all beings and all things. From this place of awareness, we put our egos and individual circumstances into proper perspective. This "Ishvara Consciousness" is cultivated through purity of body and mind, contentment with what is, the self-discipline of seeking to live our deepest beliefs as a daily practice, and through sustained spiritual studies. This is the path to focusing on the miracle of life that we experience with every breath.

Cultivating Gratitude

Just as we have the choice to become upset and reactive, we also have the choice to see all the blessings in our lives. Often, these blessings are so common and obvious that we ignore or miss them completely. What a blessing it is that the sun rises each day to shine the light of life upon Mother Earth! What a blessing Mother Earth is with her mighty rivers, mountains, forests, and valleys that nurture and sustain all life! What a blessing is the water that we drink! The food that we eat! The precious air that we breathe! What a blessing, indeed, just to be witness to all of this...to have the privilege of being alive!

I invite you to make a list right now. Write down your friends, the freedoms you enjoy, the material abundance you have, the recreational activities you enjoy, your spiritual pursuits, your freedom to speak your mind and travel at will. Don't stop there. Note all the beauty in your daily life—the flowers and birds, sunrises and sunsets, the laughter of children, and on and on.

You probably will not have time to finish this list. I don't believe you can ever finish it, because the more you ponder the blessings in life the more that will come to mind. Ultimately, everything is a blessing, even those aspects of life you have negative reactions to, because they are catalysts for change, healing, and personal growth. Everything is a blessing because it is the most profound of blessings just to be here. Just to experience the miracle of being.

The more we make these lists, even if only in our minds and hearts, the more we enter into the magical and healing realm of gratitude. Cultivating gratitude allows us, in time, to transcend our egos, our negative reactions, and the petty dramas we create for ourselves and others. Gratitude is the pathway to the Divine Being that dwells within us and the divinity that permeates the universe. With a constant sense of gratitude comes peace, contentment, bliss, and the unfolding of a whole new world before our very eyes, a world in which we live in awe of life.

To further cultivate gratitude, I invite you to say thank you to everyone and every thing. Thank you to all the ups and all the downs, and all the in-betweens. Thank you to the Divine Being that dwells within you, and thank you for the incredible privilege of life. Let us offer this thanks every day, every hour, every minute, every moment. For, all too soon, our time will pass. When that moment arrives, one of the greatest blessings we can have is knowing that we allowed ourselves to truly appreciate the journey, learned how not to sweat the small stuff, and that we knew full well what we had before it was gone.

◆ ◆ ◆ ◆ ◆ ◆ ◆ ◆ ◆ ◆

ANCIENT WISDOM
FOR
MODERN TIMES

Prajna (Illumination)

*Stay open to hearing
your inner wisdom and
following its guidance.*

Smriti (Remembering)

*Remember all moments
of illumination for they
are the wisdom of your Soul
giving you Divine guidance.*

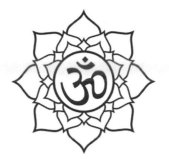

Chapter 17

What Do You Really Want?

You might be asking right about now, "Why are you telling me to 'try and try' for what I really want, when at the same time I hear you saying that I need to let go of all of my desires, that no amount of accomplishment, fortune, or fame is going to make me whole? What is it I'm supposed to really want and try to manifest if this inner revolution of Yoga is about letting go of all my wants?"

You have a good point, and it's true that I'm inviting you to let go of all your wants—your *external* wants. The *internal* is what we are after, because deep in our hearts we are all seeking the same thing: the *reclaiming of our inner power, the fullest expression of who we really are, and the lasting contentment this brings*. We all want to drink from the Rainbow Waterfall. We want the feeling of being whole, at peace with the world and ourselves, no longer fearful, anxious, or angry, but instead living in gratitude, acceptance, and loving kindness. It's in this state that our inner power shines like a torch, that we can truly experience the world, determine our role in it, live our truth, and fully express ourselves. We can't help but want this. It's our nature.

It's true that it's virtually impossible to feel content when we lack the funds to pay our rent, are in a dead-end job, or stuck in a failing relationship. It's just that resolving these problems won't bring us lasting contentment or fulfillment. Of course, it's helpful to fix these problems, but we will still be us and in no time new problems will pop up to take their place, and most of them will be of our own making. Again, no material possession, no amount of money, no promotion or enhanced prestige, *no external circumstance will give us lasting contentment or fulfillment.*

There are a million things, including what I've just mentioned, that will give us *temporary* contentment. It feels great to get a raise, have a new relationship, or buy a new possession. For a while. It feels great to eat a sumptuous meal, drink a few glasses of wine, or have a night on the town. For a while. Same thing with a vacation, an adventure, a movie, a good conversation, and so forth. They're all activities that give us a sense of pleasure, enjoyment, and relief from our stress. These aren't bad things, and we needn't forgo them. In fact, we should enjoy them. We just need to see them for what they are and make sure we don't use them as escapes, get addicted to them, or confuse them with what we are really after in life.

When we get temporary contentment from something we seek to repeat the experience because it feels so good to forget about our worries for a while. As a result, we get attached to our pleasures and distractions. This is what habituation is all about. The catch is that our pleasures are elusive, don't last, or don't always work out the way we planned. As a result, our level of contentment is always in flux, always coming and going, at risk, never really under our control. When we don't get what we think we need, or things go wrong, we feel anxious and disturbed. This is the very definition of stress.

This is also where addiction comes from. It's why so many of us become alcoholics, constant shoppers, overeaters, thrill seekers, and dependent on drugs. We're caught in an endless quest for a lasting contentment that we'll never find through these external experiences. No wonder so many of us are frustrated and feel incomplete no matter how much we achieve, how comfy and cozy our circumstances are, or how great our lives look on the surface.

Lasting contentment is only possible once we realize that we are whole just as we are, that no external situation ever will fulfill us, that there is no need to mind what is going on in our lives or worry about controlling it.

Lasting contentment comes when we live from our hearts rather than our egos, when we find who we truly are and live in alignment with the Divine Being within and with the grace of Mother Nature around us.

Lasting contentment arises from making shifts in our consciousness and changing ourselves rather than seeking to change the world so that it conforms to our illusions of how it should be.

Lasting contentment also arises from detachment.

The Power of Detachment

There's a key word here that is often misunderstood: Detachment. It can bring up visions of sticking our heads in the sand, running away to live in a cave and chanting OM all day, or letting life roll over us without standing up for ourselves. True detachment, however, means living with courage, clarity, and strength. It is living without being so hooked on our script, not trying to gratify our egos all time, or coming apart when life smacks us in the face.

It doesn't mean we have to give up our pleasures, release our ambitions, or turn away from success. We can still enjoy all the things that give us gratification and fulfillment, as long as they are not destructive addictions. Just release being attached to them. Don't let them define who you are. Remember that good times will come, they will surely go, and they will never make you whole.

Detachment also allows us to move towards our inner power because we're no longer getting stressed over everything that occurs in our lives that displeases us. We act skillfully rather than react. We accept the ever-fluctuating exigencies of life with an expanded capacity to contain, and even embrace, all that is. Reaction to life drains our power. Detachment and skillful action ignite it.

Detachment is a door we must open to enter into the realm of liberation.

Liberation is not becoming free from oppressive circumstances; it is freedom from our ego-based reactions to the events of our lives.
It is being IN the world, but not OF the world.

Being IN the world means being fully present to all the ebbs and flows of life. In this state of awareness we are more in touch with our inner wisdom and therefore more capable of making intelligent, non-emotional decisions in times of challenge and adversity. Being OF the world means we are attached...attached to the futile desire to control all outcomes, attached to our long lists of likes and dislikes, and ever fearful or angry when it seems like things are not working out exactly the way we envisioned them.

Being attached in this way is liking constructing walls around ourselves that hem us in and leave little to no opportunity for creative or intuitive expression. We begin to march through life in stiff lockstep with our preconceived ideas and ever-narrowing perspectives. When we open fully to the present moment and access our inner wisdom, we dance through life, continue to explore ourselves, find new solutions, and make discoveries about who we really are.

Detachment Practice

It takes practice to make any shift, especially shifting into detachment. Try some of the following practices and stay with the ones that resonate most with you.

- Recognize the "temporary contentments" in your life that that you have known for some time are not really in your best interest and do your best not to indulge in them. This takes great skill, so be patient with yourself.
- Practice self-acceptance. It's okay to be you, here, now, in the present moment, without anything to distract you. Detach from the impulse to do something other than just be here now.
- Feel into any anxiousness that arises. Don't run from it. Just feel into it. Notice it. Don't buy into it either.
- Remember that it's our perspective on life's chores and obligations that brings us contentment or misery, power or pain.
- Look around. Notice the sky, the birds, the trees, the flowers blossoming, the beauty of it all. It's a miracle, isn't it? What a joy to be you!

See your glass as half full because it's usually overflowing. More than half of humankind lives on less than two dollars per day. Tragically, thousands of people starve every day. Millions of us have no indoor plumbing or electricity and have never even heard of an iPod or the Internet. If we live in the First World, we have virtually everything we need, and then some. If you have food, shelter, transportation, a phone, more than one pair of shoes, and you've ever taken a vacation, your glass isn't just overflowing, it is a flood tide. The invitation here is to get excited about your life. Count your blessings. Smile. Whenever you're feeling like your glass is half empty, consider this:

> *The universe contains billions of galaxies swirling around in endless space. One galaxy is ours: the Milky*

Way. It's one hundred thousand light years in diameter, with approximately two hundred to four hundred billion stars. Near one edge of our spiraling galaxy is a tiny pinprick of light that we call our sun. One million times smaller than the sun, like a microscopic speck of dust, is our home, Earth, swirling around our sun at the speed of sixty-seven thousand miles per hour while rotating at one thousand miles per hour. Billions of times smaller than Earth, there is you...and me...and almost seven billion other humans on the planet. How tiny we are! What a cosmic ride we are on! It is utterly amazing just to be an infinitesimally small part of this never ending phantasmagoria...and the length of time we are here, in relation to the billions of years since the so-called Big Bang, is less than a snap of our fingers. Let's keep it in perspective, drop all our dramas, and get on with enjoying ourselves.

◆ ◆ ◆ ◆ ◆ ◆ ◆ ◆ ◆ ◆

ANCIENT WISDOM
FOR
MODERN TIMES

Standing in Yoga

Being fully in the moment,
completely present with yourself
and the world around you,
is standing in Yoga.

When you are fully present,
the miraculous qualities
of even the most mundane and
ordinary things are revealed,
and life becomes filled with bliss.

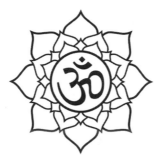

Chapter 18

Human Doings

Do you keep a constant list of things to do? As soon as you scratch one thing off your list, do you find yourself adding two or three new tasks? Maybe you even have numerous lists around the house in various places? Are you always thinking about the next activity? When you come home from a long day, do you get busy puttering around or caught up with the TV? When a moment of silence comes along, do you turn on some music, go surf the Internet or call a friend?

If you're like most of us, you do several or all of these things on a regular basis. We're always busy, on the go, rushing around, on a mission. Mentally, we're onto the next thing before we've finished the thing we're doing. It's one thing to be organized, efficient, effective and make good use of our time. It's something else to be so hooked on doing that we can't even concentrate on our current doing and we feel anxious and uncomfortable when we are not doing.

We are Human BEINGS...not Human DOINGS.

Even experienced meditation practitioners, especially those from the West, often find that their minds still spin like tops after years of practice. You can probably play your favorite sport for hours, take a long hike or sit at your computer half the day. But try to sit quietly and hold perfectly still for ten minutes. It's very challenging for most of us. The minds seems to get louder and faster. At some point, one of those things on our list of "things to do" pops up in our mind. It just won't go away. Eventually, it becomes irresistible. We can't help but jump up and take care of it, jot down a new task we just thought of, and then putter around doing something else.

We have become Human Doings, perpetually on the go, planning, strategizing, and distracting ourselves in myriad ways. This incessant turbulence in our lives muddies the waters of our consciousness. It disenfranchises us from the present moment. It makes true relaxation virtually impossible. It's like having the engine of our car on all the time, even when it's parked in our garage...which is a formula for wearing out all its parts and running out of gas.

> *To bring harmony into our lives, we must seek to become Human BEINGS once again and let go of our constant doing.*
>
> *The only place we find true contentment is in the state of Pure Being.*
>
> *The only place we find true compassion in the state of Pure Being.*
>
> *The only place we find true healing in the state of Pure Being.*
>
> *The only place we find true self-awareness in the state of Pure Being.*
>
> *The only place we can connect with our hearts in the state of Pure Being.*

The only place we become true Human Beings in the state of Pure Being.

To begin a journey into the Pure Being, we first need to slow down. It's not so easy, and doing it abruptly can be dangerous to our health. There are many examples of highly driven, very successful, seemingly healthy, Type A people who retire early and die shortly thereafter. Their entire identity was wrapped up in their high-powered careers, and without all that doing—which served them very well in the workplace—they just didn't know what to do with themselves. More accurately, they didn't know how to "not do." This increases stress and tension, blood pressure rises, hearts fail. Unfortunately, it happens all the time.

Slowing down and slipping into the state of Pure Being is a subtle art that can't be forced, and it's an art few of us are ever taught. From early on, we learn to do and do and do, and to feel inadequate and incomplete if we are not doing. It becomes our identity, and it forms our relationship with the world around us. It's as if we are always racing against time, convinced the more we can jam-pack into each day, the better our lives will be. This is why it's called the Rat Race.

A Rat Race is defined as "A fierce competition to maintain or improve one's position in the workplace or in social life." It also suggests an endless, self-defeating, or pointless pursuit. The analogy is to a laboratory rat trying to escape by running around in the little exercise wheel in its cage...and, of course, getting nowhere.

There is growing national awareness that working long hours, putting in overtime, commuting, and having less time for our family and friends is a recipe for unhappiness and illness. Millions of people in the rat race find they cannot even enjoy their increased prosperity because they don't know how to stop running around in the wheel. They feel caged. They are caged. It's a trap. It's proof that more money, more material acquisitions, more prestige, and more accomplishments don't translate into more bliss...in truth, it's just the opposite.

Even if we aren't global corporate execs, holding down three jobs, or commuters working overtime, most of us are busy creating our own versions of the Rat Race. Running around in circles winds us up tightly (this is why we feel "uptight") and pumps more adrenalin through our bodies. We get addicted to this cycle of doing. Every day we jump back on the wheel without even noticing it and begin the spin all over again.

> *To heal and transform, we need to leave the rat race and rejoin the Human Race...not the Human Doing Race, but the Human Being Race.*

In a word, all this doing is excess. Excess is the root cause of human imbalance, illness, and suffering. One-third of all Americans are overweight, and more than half of them are considered obese. This is a staggering statistic and at the core of our health care crisis. This contributes to current epidemics of diabetes, cancer, heart attack, stroke and other major, life-threatening illnesses.

> *Excess equals imbalance.*

> *Imbalance equals suffering.*

> *Moderation equals balance.*

> *Balance equals healing.*

A sizable majority Americans suffer from what we might call "external obesity." Take a peek in your closets, cupboards, garage, and storage spaces. Look at all that stuff you never use. Like too much weight in your body, it bogs you down. We are so attached to all our stuff, however, that it's a struggle to toss out or give away things we haven't used in years. This excess has global implications as well. It takes an inordinate amount of the finite resources of our planet to make all the stuff we have.

The good news is that we can lighten our load, and in doing so we will feel a sense of freedom and spaciousness in our lives.

Moderation Practice

Moderation is gentle pathway towards become Human Beings rather than Human Doings. Consider the following suggestions:

- Do less. Cut out all the things on your list that aren't really vital.
- Try to sit in stillness and silence for a few minutes each day, even if your mind is racing away and you start to feel itchy all over.
- Consume less. This means less food, fewer material acquisitions, fewer experiences.
- Give your stuff away. Go ahead, just do it! Clean out all your spaces and give away or toss out everything you don't really need. Don't find someone you know and give it to them...this just makes their "stuff body" more obese. Give it to charity, or simply get rid of it. During this process, when you find yourself clinging to stuff you haven't used in years, just laugh out loud at yourself, close your eyes, and put it in the goodbye pile.

You might wonder what giving your stuff away has to do with becoming more of a Human Being and less of a Human Doing. Having too much stuff is directly associated with too much doing. Part of constant doing is making trips to the mall to buy stuff we don't need. You will also find that it is an amazing emotional detoxification. You'll feel lighter and healthier. There is a subtle dignity and elegance to the process. You'll be proud of yourself, and you'll feel much more like a Human Being...guaranteed.

❖ ❖ ❖ ❖ ❖ ❖ ❖ ❖ ❖ ❖

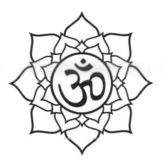

Chapter 19
Miracles

What time did you wake up this morning? From that time until now, if it's only been a few minutes or a few hours, there have been untold miracles occurring all around you. Every day, from the moment we first awaken, the Universe is showering us with miracles. We're surrounded by them. It's like a rainbow waterfall cascading over us, washing us with grace. There are so many miracles on any given day that it would be impossible to list them all in a single book. It would take volumes and volumes, and still there would be more. Funny, though, we miss out on most of them because we don't even know they are there.

Why do we fail to see them? Most of us immediately begin distracting ourselves in the morning. We click on the TV or radio, go online, grab the newspaper, or simply get lost again in our busy minds. Or we jump out of bed and quickly get going. There's so much to do, plans to make, places to be, things to be accomplished. I'm not saying there's anything inherently wrong with this. We need to plan our lives, get things done, accomplish this and that. The problem is that we become so consumed with distracting ourselves or with constant doing that we miss what's going on around us. We miss the eternal moment. We blind ourselves to the simple miracles of being alive.

When we can't see or experience how amazing the world around is, and forget what a privilege it is to be alive, we get caught up in our worries, apprehensions, angers, and fears. It's easier to become cynical, forlorn, negative, and depressed. This makes us even more alienated from the present moment, more insulated from the miracles all around us, more caught up in our stuff.

Even if we are aware of the concept of miracles and fully agree with it, we forget. When we forget life loses a great deal of its luster. Artificial stimuli take the place of the true blessings around us, and these unnatural experiences never truly satisfy. The good news is that it only takes one thing to completely reconnect with the miracle of being: attention. All we need to do is to pay attention.

Attention is the key to Presence.

Presence is the key to Awareness.

Awareness brings Consciousness.

Consciousness opens our eyes to Miracles.

Opening to Simple Miracles

The first breath you took when you woke up today was a miracle. So was every subsequent breath, and so is the next breath you are about to take. It's the most precious gift you can experience. Each breath is an affirmation of your existence, an empowerment, a drinking in of the nectar of life itself. Pause for a moment, right now, and drink in a deep and full, slow and smooth breath. Notice how it feels, how it tastes inside, how its essence permeates your entire being. Remember what an amazing gift of life it is to breathe. Have profound gratitude for this. Feel the miracle.

Take a sip of water. All the raindrops and rivers and waterfalls of Mother Earth are giving you this amazing gift. That water was once in the ocean, once in snowcapped mountains, once in a mighty river. Eons ago it may have been sipped by dinosaurs or absorbed by great forests. Perhaps Jesus drank that water, or Buddha, Mother Theresa, or Mahatma Gandhi. Now it is merging with you. You are becoming that.

Notice the sky. Whether it's cloudy or clear, it is a miraculous sight. Feel the breeze on your face, notice the temperature of the morning, stretch your arms and legs...it's all a miracle, and you yourself are a unique and amazing miracle of life as well.

As the famed naturalist John Muir said, "When we try to pick out anything by itself, we find it hitched to everything else in the Universe."

The Miracle of Now

Just as we only make connection with our deeper self when we are fully in the present moment, all miracles exist in the *now*. They aren't concepts, figments of our imagination, or things of the past or future. If we are not fully present to the circumstances of our daily lives, not fully in the current time and space of wherever we happen to be, we have no connection with our deeper self or with the miracles that abound around us.

Ironically, we don't have to be in the present moment to notice our worries, our hurts, our dramas, or our wants. So, these tend to take central stage in our lives. As a result, we miss the untold blessings of being us while we connect with the misery of being us. This isn't a formula for great joy. Worrying is like praying for what we don't want...or as the great American author Samuel Clemens (aka Mark Twain) said, "I have known a great many troubles, most of which never happened." The more our mind is filled with our troubles, the more our troubles are likely to manifest in our lives. Even if our troubles never come to pass, we are poisoning ourselves with stress hormones as if they did. Does it make any sense to you to live this way?

Praying for what we DO want is a much better idea. We want energy following our best intentions, not our worst fears. What is more important, however, is coming to realize that having too many positive wants can be a trap as well, even if our intentions are worthy and noble. If we create too many new intentions and desires, we are just playing the escape game again and forgetting how many blessings are already in our lives. One or two focused intentions at a time are much better, and we should make these once we are in touch with our Divine Self, because, as I've noted, it's important to be careful about what we ask for...just in case we get it.

> *Gratitude is the pathway to fully perceiving, embracing and enjoying the miracles in our lives.*

This is another big shift: going from worry to gratitude, embracing all situations and experiences with thankfulness. The greatest miracle is that we are here, in this body, on this planet, experiencing the grace of being alive. Think about it. The alternative to being here is not being here.

Planet Earth

The planet on which we live sustains and nourishes us in a multitude of ways. It is an awesome miracle. Look around. Everything comes from Mother Earth. Not just the plants, animals, forests, mountains, valleys, rivers, and oceans, but all the stuff we industrious humans have created for our survival, comfort, and progress. Our homes, our cars, our clothing, all our possessions, our cities—everything is a gift from her. The food we eat, the water we drink, the air we breathe...all a gift, like mother's milk from her sacred breast. She gives us so much, and most of the time we just take it for granted, don't we? How can we ever express enough gratitude?

Let's consider water again. Water is one of those pervasive miracles we come in touch with every day. It supports and nourishes all life. No water means no you, no me, no us, no anything. Try remembering this every time you have an interaction with water. Do this for just one day and notice how profound it can be. Say, "Thank you," when you take a sip of water (or anything else because all liquids we drink are water-based), when you run the tap to clean a dish, turn on the shower, or flush the toilet, say, "thank you," to

Mother Earth. If it rains, or you are by a river or jump into a pool, say, "Thank you!"

Then there's the air. What a great, miraculous gift it is to experience the air! Pay close attention to every breath, with the awareness of what a miracle it is to interact with the air this way. No breath equals no you, no me, no us, no anything. Listen to the whisper of the breeze, notice how the trees sway, watch clouds float by in the sky. Say, "Thank you!"

Go outside during the day, look up and glimpse the sun. Feel its warmth pouring into you. Think of the fire it gives us, with which we cook our food, warm our homes, light our world. The heat in your body, your digestive juices, and your neurological system contain fire from the sun. Its life force is inside of you. Contemplate how flowers open their petals and reach towards the sun, drinking in life from its radiance while exhaling exotic fragrances. They create vegetables and fruits that we savor and ingest into our beings. No sun equals no you, no me, no us, no anything. Say, "Thank you!"

Fix your gaze on anything...any little thing. If you give it the chance, it will bewilder you. Let yourself be bewildered all the time. Find your inner child, that precious being who saw the magic in everything...in your first rainbow, a frog hopping in a pond, a hummingbird sipping at a blossom, the stars splashed in the night sky, raindrops on your tongue. It's all still miraculous. Everything. Even a weed pushing up through a crack in the cement, mold growing on stale bread, a bug beneath a rock. Miracles!

If you're indoors, gaze at the first thing you see and contemplate where it came from. All of its components will reveal themselves as miracles. Take this book that you are holding in your hands. It's pages came from trees. Those trees were nourished by sun and water and soil. The elements of earth, water, and fire are in your hands as you hold this. Astonishing, isn't it?

This is *attention,* it is coming into the present moment and seeing the Divine expressing itself all around us. Attention cannot help but promote gratitude and bring us from that busy place in our heads down to that deep and eternal place in our hearts. It aligns us with the Divine every time. It is the shift that lies at the core of all spiritual practice and the key to personal transformation.

Awareness and gratitude are pathways to contentment, acceptance, peace, loving kindness, and Self-realization.

There are five elements that comprise all that is: earth, water, fire, air, and space. Each element is a miracle. Not only are these miraculous elements everywhere in our world, they are *within* us. Your bones, tissues, and organs are earth. Every cell of your body is also mostly water. Our internal fire warms us and digests our food. Air courses through us and feeds our life force. Our inner space, like a universe itself, contains all this.

You are that. You are Mother Earth and she is You. You are the Sun and he is you. You are Spirit and Spirit is you. You are eternally connected in the most elemental and universal of ways to all that is. The more you can open this, the more you hold this connection in your awareness and in your hearts, the more you live the essence of Vedic Wisdom and Deep Yoga.

Nature is the greatest medicine, the greatest healer, the greatest embodiment of consciousness and the present moment.

Even though everything comes from Mother Earth, the environments we create with her abundance are largely artificial and unbalancing. Spend an entire day in a busy city or staring at a computer screen and you feel frazzled. End that day in nature watching the sunset and you feel replenished and restored. This amazing medicine doesn't cost a dime. There are no side effects. You can't overdose on the sunset or the sunrise. Go for it. You'll be glad you did.

Treasure Hunt

Remember when you were a child how fun treasure hunts were? Become a Miracle Hunter. Look for them everywhere. After you notice the most obvious ones, look for the hidden ones. See miracles in the smallest, most ordinary things. Notice how you feel each time you find one.

Cultivate deep gratitude towards these miracles. Thank them for being in your life. Thank your food before you eat it for supporting your time here on Mother Earth. Thank Mother Earth every time you take a step, lie down, or breathe her in. Thank your miraculous heart for beating, your eyes for seeing, your fingers for touching, your ears for hearing, your nose for smelling, your tongue for tasting.

Write down five or ten of your favorite miracles and post them somewhere. Peek at that list now and then as a reminder of what a joy it is to be you, what a privilege it is to experience such miraculous things. This is the practice of standing in Yoga, expanding your consciousness, and transforming your life.

◆ ◆ ◆ ◆ ◆ ◆ ◆ ◆ ◆ ◆

ANCIENT WISDOM
FOR
MODERN TIMES

OM

OM is the sound of all creation.

It is the beginning, middle and the end of it all or the past, present and future.

Chanting OM connects you with the inner rhythms of your body, breath and consciousness.

It is a prayer to the oneness of all that is.

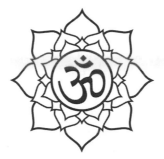

Chapter 20

Edging Through

The summer before my fifth birthday, my father surprised me with a new bicycle. I was still using trainer wheels on my first bike to stabilize its twelve-inch wheels. I had come to biking late in my childhood since I was stricken by polio at three years old and was in a leg brace with a corrective shoe for more than a year. The new bike, shiny and silver with sixteen-inch wheels, looked gigantic. It was exciting and frightening at the same time. I watched with apprehension as my father removed the trainer wheels from my old bike and put them on the new one. Before I knew it, he hoisted me onto the seat. My feet dangled a few inches above the ground. Looking down, I felt like I was on top of a tall building.

"By your birthday," my father said, "we'll take those trainer wheels off and you'll ride this bike all by yourself like a big boy."

That's when I freaked out. We had tried this with my small bike months earlier, and I had fallen right over. I hit the street hard and lay there crying for several minutes, mostly from fear that I had disappointed my daddy. Now, I could see myself tumbling from the high seat of this much bigger bike and crashing harder. The pavement below me looked like it was licking its lips, just waiting to chew up my elbows and knees, or even break an arm or a leg. Worse, I thought, I'll disappoint my daddy again, I won't ever be a "big boy."

For the next several months as my birthday approached, I was never able to enjoy that beautiful new bike. Every time I climbed onto it and pedaled along, I thought about the looming *Day of Judgment* when my trusted trainer wheels would be removed. The crashes I visualized in my mind became worse and worse—broken bones, head split open, an ambulance rushing to the scene with sirens blaring and taking me away as my father stood there with his arms tightly crossed, shaking his head in disappointment at my failure while all the neighborhood children looked on shaking their heads at what a wimp I was.

My birthday came the week before school began, and as it approached I knew the dreaded day would soon arrive. A few days before this moment of reckoning over which I had become so emotionally worked up, I decided to take action. I began telling myself there was nothing to fear and that I really could do it. It was a tough sell, but as I rode my bike each day I began experimenting by building up some speed and then coasting, noticing which training wheel was hitting the pavement to keep me upright. I would then try to center the bike and lift it off the training wheel on that side. When I overcompensated and felt the opposite training wheel hit the pavement, I would do my best to bring the bike back to center again. Occasionally, often when I least expected it, I would find that groove and be able to keep the bike off both training wheels for increasingly longer periods of time.

Next, I started tackling the bigger problem: My fears. Whenever they would arise, with all the visions of crashing and burning, I would try to face them squarely and see myself cycling along at top speed with no trainer wheels like a professional bike racer. It was a struggle, but I kept at it as best as a soon-to-be five year old could until the big day finally arrived. Even though it was so long ago, I can still recall the warm Sunday morning with clear blue skies. Our quiet suburban street looked beautiful with all the lawns neatly trimmed and flowers in bloom in front of the small stucco houses. I summoned all my newfound courage, but as my father removed the trainer wheels it was like my last security blanket was being taken away and I felt a lump in my throat.

"I'll run next to you and keep you from falling until you get the hang of it," my father said as he lifted me onto the seat. "Your feet don't touch the ground," he added, "so be sure to slide forward off the seat when you stop and get your feet on the ground."

I don't think I really understood his instructions. In truth, I was hardly listening. My heart was pounding as adrenalin raced through my veins. I secretly hoped that an ambulance really was close by to whisk me away, especially before any of the other kids on the block witnessed my humiliating downfall. I swallowed hard and did my best to erase that vision and see myself riding with the greatest of ease, but the lump in my throat wouldn't go away.

Suddenly, we were off. True to his word, my father was running beside me with one hand on the back of the seat and the other gently on my shoulder. "Here we go," he said after a few dozen yards, "you can do it!"

As I gained speed, my dad let go. I was shaky for a few seconds and then, suddenly, I slipped into a place of awareness I had never consciously experienced. Everything seemed like slow-motion. All sounds stopped. The street looked wider and felt smoother than ever. The houses around me seemed to disappear. It was just me, cruising on top of that big bike. I could feel my weight distributed perfectly, the balance felt elegant, and it was effortless. All my fears and apprehensions vanished as I took full command. The adrenalin melted away and was replaced by a warm inner river of joy and self-empowerment. The smile on my face was almost reaching my ears.

I finally circled to return, and as the world around me reappeared I could hear my dad cheering me on. "Atta boy! Atta boy!" I rode right up to him, hit the breaks and jumped forward off the seat, landing both feet on the pavement and keeping the bike upright. I had done it! It was a breakthrough I would never forget. Every time I got on that bike again I took off like a rocket, making up time for the year I missed with polio. As I screamed down the street, I wondered why I had ever been so worried and thought about all the time I had wasted that summer being in fear and feeling incapable.

Releasing False Agreements

This type of self-created suffering over something that never happens is a common problem. We often make false agreements with ourselves that we don't have what it takes to chart the course of our lives. We create illusory limitations and hang onto past experiences, real or imagined, that keep us from moving forward. This creates what Yoga calls *samskaras*, or impressions, real or imagined, that get etched into our subconscious.

When I first fell off my smaller bike without the trainer wheels, I created a samskara. Unknowingly, I held onto it deeply in my subconscious. I couldn't being to consider ever taking those support wheels off my bike again. When my father turned up with the bigger bike, my fear boiled over beyond all reason. My anxiety deepened as I "horrible-ized" over the potential consequences of repeating the fall. Fortunately, with a little introspection, I was able to make a shift, and I experienced an important lesson in self-empowerment in the process.

Deeper samskaras arise from more traumatic life experiences, such as a death in the family, a terrible accident, the loss of our job, or separation from our partner. They also come from repeated negative experiences, such as an angry or drunken parent regularly showering verbal abuse on a young child or a soldier witnessing repeated violence in combat and ending up with Post Traumatic Stress Disorder. Many of us also unknowingly condition ourselves to overreact to minor events in our lives that our subconscious connects to the larger events that traumatized us earlier.

Letting Go of Old Agreements

As we enter our adult lives, we often have a multiplicity of these samskaras. Unless we learn to let them go, we become increasingly stressed out, fearful, angry, limited, and reactive. This creates a pattern of getting uptight about a variety of life experiences and circumstances that are inherently insignificant. It's little wonder we sometimes find ourselves in situations where we know we are overreacting but we are incapable of controlling our responses. Our higher self witnesses our lower self acting out in embarrassing fashion, and yet the higher self can't seem intervene. This patterning leads to mental imbalances and, ultimately, more serious problems.

Yoga and Ayurveda hold that behind most of the physical ailments that we face in our lives we can find a cause, or major contributing factor, deep within our minds. We can also use these sciences to reprogram ourselves, release old mental agreements and reactive patterns, and move towards healing and wholeness. Yoga poses not only make our bodies more flexible, balanced, and powerful, they also facilitate the expansion, balancing, and strengthening of our emotional bodies.

For instance, in poses such as *Parsvottanasana* (Intense Side Stretch), *Paschimottanansa* (Seated Forward Bend), *Supta Padangusthasana* (Reclining Big Toe Pose), *Trikonasana* (Triangle Pose) and *Uttanasa* (standing forward Bend), we deeply stretch our hamstrings and open our hips. When we are first introduced to such asanas, we often find ourselves tensing up and recoiling from the extreme sensations we experience in the areas most affected by these poses.

What we are really feeling is fear. This fear triggers the tension. The tension, in turn, makes our muscles resistant to expanding. We are now incapable of moving deeper into the pose, and we have increased the possibility of injury. But as we learn to breathe more deeply and relax in our practice, things begin to change. We become more able to accept the challenging sensations. Our fear dissipates. Our muscles and tendons expand and become more supple. Our *prana*, or life force, begins to flow more freely. We advance in the posture and feel empowered.

The same holds true for our life experiences. If we can apply this process off our mats and relax more deeply into our lives, practicing acceptance, expanding our range, and releasing our fears, we can open to a wider range of circumstances and challenges. We then pattern ourselves to act more skillfully and, most importantly, to react less. Our samskaras are reduced, or at least they no longer run the show all the time. We can then begin to meditate on our deep-seated fears and painful memories as we create new relationships with ourselves and the world around us. Through this process we begin to heal, become empowered, and begin to transform our lives.

Finding the Edge

As a practice, I invite you to choose a few Yoga poses that you find the most challenging, especially in the areas of hips and hamstrings. Begin to perform them on a regular basis, daily if possible. Be gentle with yourself, but also find the "edge" in each pose: that place where you would usually back out. Stay in the pose without forcing it. Hold it two or even three times longer than you normally would. Breathe more deeply. Become more present. Experience all sensations without any judgment or aversion. Relax, let go, and just be with it.

You might feel a little bit sore at first, but some long, hot baths will take care of this. With dedication to this practice, you will soon find yourself opening more deeply in your poses, feeling accomplished, and experiencing greater benefits from your Yoga. Your muscles will feel more supple. Your prana will be more vibrant. You might even feel deep emotional releases as old memories and tensions begin to dissolve.

Then, practice these acceptance, relaxation, and release techniques off your mat and in your daily life whenever old, habituated, negative responses or inner agreements arise. See them for what they are, and then create an affirmation—a positive statement to silently repeat to yourself that affirms you. For instance, if you were traumatized by a strict parent and it has stuck with you and caused feelings of anger and insecurity, you might say to yourself, "The past is over. I am at peace and courageously living in the present moment." If you tend to get angry quickly over little things, you might repeat, "I am choosing peace." All our experiences and samskaras are unique, but in time you will find the right words to act as antidotes that works for you.

With devoted and regular practice, emotional mountains will dwindle down into molehills. You will react to challenges less often and act skillfully more often. There will be less drama in your life and more clarity. You will have found your groove, moved past your samskaras, and relaxed through the "edge," to a more positive place in your life.

◆ ◆ ◆ ◆ ◆ ◆ ◆ ◆ ◆ ◆

ANCIENT WISDOM
FOR
MODERN TIMES

Mauna

Mauna is silence.

The silence of pure presence
and pure awareness.

The silence of your inner landscape.

The unspoken voice of
consciousness within you.

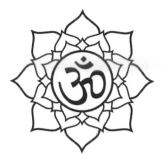

Chapter 20
Laugh It Off

Laughing in the face of death is an old cliche, but one that a courageous man proved to be true. Norman Cousins bucked the medical establishment, literally laughed in the face of death, and prevailed. Cousins was a renowned journalist, author, editor, publisher, and peace activist who stunned the world back in the 1980s. At the pinnacle of his career, he was diagnosed with a rare arthritic disease that often proved fatal. He was in terrible pain and his chances of survival were dim. Mainstream medicine had little to offer him except palliative medicine: painkillers, muscle relaxants, and antidepressants to mask his symptoms.

At one point in his multifaceted career, Cousins had served as Adjunct Professor of Medical Humanities for the School of Medicine at the University of California, Los Angeles, where he had conducted research on the biochemistry of human emotions. During his studies, he was fascinated by the overwhelming scientific evidence suggesting that negative thinking had a direct correlation to illness.

In seeking to deal with his own health crisis, he hypothesized that if a bad attitude created a toxic biochemistry, a good attitude should create a healing biochemistry. Putting his theory into action, he checked out of the hospital and into a first class hotel, where he and his wife watched Marx Brother comedy movies and laughed like crazy. Cousins focused on cultivating a positive attitude of faith, love, and hope to go with the laughter.

He soon found his theory was panning out. When his pain flared up, ten minutes of belly laughter alone miraculously anesthetized him for a few hours and allowed some desperately needed sleep. Upon awakening, when the pain came back, he flicked on more movies, laughed heartily some more, and—just like magic—the pain subsided again. According to Cousins, it worked every time. He overcame his agony without all the drugs his doctors had prescribed and, ultimately, he self-healed.

The medical establishment dismissed Cousins' experience as a fluke, characterized his laughter and positive attitude practices as ridiculous and suggested he may not have been so sick in the first place. Over the next several decades, however, scientific research proved what Cousins had hypothesized and eventually he became heralded as one of the pioneers of modern mind/body medicine.

This was the very alchemy of cultivating positive emotions that Yoga prescribes. Cousins was using his brain to make neurochemicals that relieved his pain, allowing him to relax and heal. In doing so, he illustrated that we really do have the capacity to take charge of our minds, shift our attitudes, and transform our lives.

All obstacles are blessings in disguise.

All suffering is an opportunity for healing and transformation.

Cousins also illustrated how a circumstance that most of us would perceive as a huge negative can be a great blessing. Not only did he face death and win, he inspired others to try healing laughter, and many of them formed groups to share Cousins' techniques with wider audiences. This helped thousands of people make a shift, take charge, and tap into their inner healing power.

Of course, not all of us can laugh our way out of life-threatening disease, but it will surely enhance our chances to improve or deal with our condition. Even if we're not critically ill, laughter can help us heal in many ways. When we laugh, we take ourselves less seriously. We forget about our worries. We forget about our egos. Whatever walls we have put up around ourselves come tumbling down.

Something seems to happen to so many of us as we get older. We forget how to laugh...to really laugh, the art of just letting it all go. This is part of losing touch with our inner child. For some of us, it even seems embarrassing to go crazy with laughter. We don't want to make spectacles of ourselves or do anything outside of the boundaries of what we feel is socially acceptable. Ironically, it seems more socially acceptable to go crazy with anger and make a scene than to let our guard down and laugh!

Laughing helps you to heal.

Laughing brings you into the present moment.

Laughing makes you feel good.

Laughing dissolves your stress.

The biggest shift is to learn to laugh at yourself.

We take ourselves too seriously most of the time, don't we? For the most part, it doesn't get us where we want to be. I'm not suggesting that you go around being silly all day long, laughing uproariously at everything and everyone. I'm suggesting a little levity now and then, and that you find some time to really let it all go, where and when it feels appropriate.

When you've done this just a few times, you'll be imprinted: You'll remember how good it feels, and you'll be more able to access this state of mind with ease. In other words, you can conjure up an inner, silent laugh at times when you may have otherwise reacted with a negative attitude. When you do slip and have a needlessly bad reaction to something (which you *will* do—we ALL do this), just have an inner chuckle about it as well. You'll find it helps you to digest and release the experience and move on from there.

Laughter brings us fully into the present moment, that place where we can't even remember our worries.It creates positive neurotransmitters, including serotonin, a neurochemical that influences a variety of our psychological and bodily functions. It not only dissolves our aches and pains, it affects most of the approximately forty-million cells in our brain. This includes brain cells related to mood, sexual desire and function, appetite, sleep, memory and learning, body temperature regulation, and social behavior. Serotonin also affects the functioning of our cardiovascular system, our muscles, and various elements of our endocrine system. Low levels of serotonin are associated with anxiety disorders, panic attacks, excess anger and depression.

The point is that we have a choice, a conscious choice at every turn. We can react to circumstances, or we can act skillfully. We can poison ourselves, or we can be more relaxed in dealing with what sets us off. Anger harms you, laughter heals you. Which do you choose? Makes you want to laugh, doesn't it? Go ahead, have at it right now.

Laugh It Off!

- Find time to have a big belly laugh at least once a day. Really let it out! Sustain this for a few minutes, then notice how you feel. If you pay really close attention, you'll experience the sensation of soothing serotonin inside of you.
- Laugh at yourself on a regular basis, even if it's just a silent, inner laugh.
- Laugh when your ego kicks up, when you are irrational, when you get cranky, and when you get angry.
- Smile a lot. It's just like a subtle laugh and easier to get away with in public.

◆ ◆ ◆ ◆ ◆ ◆ ◆ ◆ ◆ ◆

ANCIENT WISDOM
FOR
MODERN TIMES

Jai Ma (Victory to the Mother)

Jai Ma!
May the Divine Feminine prevail!
Victory to the forces of
peace, creation, nurturing,
and sustaining.

Jai Ma!
May we ever worship
the Divine Mother in all
her manifestations!

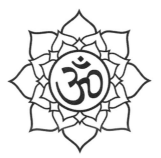

Chapter 21

Honoring the
Divine Mother

"May there only be peaceful and cheerful earth days to come for our beautiful Spaceship Earth as it continues to spin and circle in frigid space with its warm and fragile cargo of animate life."

~United Nations Secretary General U Thant, Burmese diplomat, March 21, 1971, on the occasion of the first international recognition of Earth Day.

There is a growing global awareness about the importance of protecting the earth, being more mindful about our stewardship of the environment, and deciding what we can do as individuals to make a contribution to this effort. Every spring, millions of people around the world celebrate Earth Day. Still, we lose our focus and we forget. Car engines are kept running at the drive-up windows at the bank or while waiting to pick up children at school. We over-consume. Forget to recycle. Buy things we don't really need. Spend too long in the shower. Allow the grocery clerk to pack our things in plastic bags because it was too inconvenient to bring bags from home.

It's not that we are evil, we just forget. The stress and fast pace of our daily lives takes over and we fall into our daily patterns and lose awareness. We are also often unaware of subtle ways in which we might be harming our planet. The contents and packaging of products we buy may contain toxic substances that we have overlooked. Our food and clothing may come from corporations who exploit third world environments and societies. Our investments in mutual funds may include holdings in companies that plunder and pollute with reckless abandon. We just don't see it unless we are vigilant. It is far easier to feel anger towards the obvious exploiters and polluters of the world, towards those who wage war and are inhumane, than to see ourselves and be aware of any small contributions we might be making to harming Mother Earth. Yet true change doesn't begin with protesting the actions of others, it starts with changing our own lives.

The Vedic wisdom of Yoga and its sister science of Ayurveda offer us several pathways into greater remembrance and personal transformation. From a Vedic viewpoint, the earth is much more than a spaceship revolving in the cosmos. She is Mother Earth, a manifestation of the Divine. We are much more than passengers on an impersonal planet, we are manifestations of the Mother and embodiments of the Divine. We are Mother Earth and she is us. This isn't just a metaphysical idea or a New Age notion. You really are her, and she really is you.

Ayurveda, the holistic medical system that arose from the Vedas, views the physical body, and all of nature, as composed of the *mahabhutas*, or five elements of earth, air, fire, water, and space. Mother Earth is the womb from which these elements arise, and to which they return in the elegant cycle of life and death. Every cell in your body is composed of these five elements. All the food, even the nourishment provided to you in the womb and the mother's milk you drank, came from Mother Earth. Everything you have ingested to sustain since you were born came from her as well, even adulterated, processed, and junk food products come from the earth. Where else could they come from? Mars?

From the Yogic and Ayurvedic points of view, the choices we make about what we eat, and the relationship we cultivate with nature through our diet, are essential components of personal transformation and spiritual practice. Further, our very lives depend upon the intelligence of these choices. The impact of the Western Diet on global warming, world hunger, our polluted waterways, and the plight of the rainforest is equally as alarming as its effect on our health.

For instance, every minute, up to fifty acres of rainforest is cut or burned to the ground. Most of it is for grazing cattle. For every hamburger, fifty-five square feet of rainforest is destroyed. The leading cause of deforestation and species extinction worldwide is livestock grazing. Twenty-five percent of the methane produced in the world comes from livestock. Methane and carbon dioxide are the leading causes of global warming. Along with methane, one hundred fifty pounds of carbon dioxide is released into the atmosphere for every hamburger that is made. This is twenty-five times more carbon dioxide than you would release into the atmosphere by driving your car all day long.

Thirty percent of the pollution in our American waterways comes from livestock farming. The production of one pound of beef requires 2,500 gallons of water. The production of one pound of wheat or potatoes requires only 815 gallons. If we all ate a predominantly vegetarian diet we would reverse the pollution and loss of this precious resource. What is more important, we could save innocent lives. World hunger organizations estimate that fifteen million children die each year from starvation and hunger related diseases. This is forty-thousand children every day. Yet each day the world produces enough grain to provide every person on Earth with more than two loaves of bread. Forty percent of that grain, however, is fed to livestock, which means that 1.4 billion people could be fed by the grain given to U.S. livestock alone. If we reduced our meat consumption by just ten percent, we could feed every starving child on Earth if we chose to.

Awakening to how our dietary decisions not only affect our personal health, but have an impact on all of humankind and on Mother Earth, provides us deeper insight to the intricate and delicate fabric of life. To love and honor Mother Earth, we must love and honor our bodies as physical manifestations of her grace. By eating junk food and the products of factory farms, we not only support companies who exploit the environment, we harm and pollute the mother by harming and polluting ourselves. Eating fresh, organic, and locally produced food does more than promote good health, it's social activism for Mother Earth. Since we are her, and she is us, any way in which we purify ourselves helps to purify her as well.

Going with the Flow

Ayurveda also beckons us to align our lives with the rhythms of nature as a pathway to healing, inner balance, and personal growth. It recommends that we awaken at sunrise, honor the sunset, take time to get outside and drink in the moon and stars at night. It asks us to observe the seasons, and to realize that we are an integral part of these eternal cycles. This brings us into deeper harmony with the sacredness of Mother Earth and the sacredness of our individual lives as well. In modern medical terms we would call this achieving homeostasis. As we spend more time immersing ourselves in nature, we spend less time in the more unconscious pursuits of over-acquiring, over-consuming, and being manipulated by our mass-marketing culture. This, too, is social and spiritual activism.

A central ethical principle of Yoga is *ahimsa*, or non-harming. Violence and war cause the greatest harm to Mother Earth and humankind, while peace is the greatest medicine possible. A sustained and devoted practice of ahimsa includes a commitment to healing ourselves, healing humankind, and helping to protect and heal Mother Earth. Beyond not engaging in war and violence, we embrace ahimsa through mindful speech, right action towards others, being of service, and cultivating humility. Even the simple act of stooping to retrieve someone else's litter and depositing it in a garbage can is an act of practicing ahimsa.

Yoga also teaches us to transcend the ego and understand that it is not all about us. An awareness of, and alignment with, the divinity of Mother Earth is central to this process. As we come to understand that she and we are one, we realize that we are much more than our egos, our bodies, or our minds. We are connected to something much greater than our individuated selves. We are ultimately connected to all that is.

Connecting with Mother Earth

As a meditative practice to cultivate a personal connection with Mother Earth, find a quiet place to lie down, perhaps outside in nature on a warm day when possible, and close your eyes. As you allow your body and mind to let go and completely relax, feel the support beneath you. It might be the grass in a park, a meadow in the wilderness, or a sandy beach.

After a few gentle breaths, take your awareness of this support all the way to the core of Mother Earth. See that molten core as her heart. Then visualize a golden flame, like a candle flame, at your heart center right behind your breastbone. As you breathe in, take a thread of golden light from her heart into yours. As you exhale, send your light back to her heart.

When this connection is fully established, deepen your breath in a gentle and smooth way. Inhale and feel the light of Mother Earth growing brighter, filling your entire body, permeating every cell of your being. Exhale and feel your light filling Mother Earth, luminous and radiant, permeating every cell of her being. As you continue, open yourself to the experience of your oneness with nature, the sacredness of your Spirit merging with the spirit of Mother Earth. Know that you and she are one, and that you are a manifestation of her.

Let this practice remind you that every day is Earth Day. Every day is an opportunity to give thanks to Mother Earth and honor her through honoring yourself. Every day offers the renewed chance to make a contribution to the wellness of Mother Earth. Every day is an invitation to open your heart and mind to the wonder and oneness of all that is. This is the essence of Yoga.

◆ ◆ ◆ ◆ ◆ ◆ ◆ ◆ ◆ ◆ ◆

ANCIENT WISDOM
FOR
MODERN TIMES

MAUNA

Mauna is silence.

In silence we become more present.
The whisper of our Soul can then be heard.

Nature reveals her miracles to us.
The grace of being unfolds.

In silence we find
the song of life.

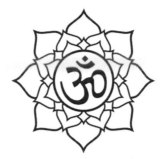

Chapter 23

The Power of Ritual

Our thoughts lead to our actions.
Our actions create our habits.
Our habits form our character.
Our character determines our destiny.

This insightful saying can be sourced back to the wisdom of the Vedas, the ancient scripts from which the practices of Yoga and Ayurveda arise. As with most Vedic Wisdom, it is elegant in its simplicity yet profoundly deep and complex as we contemplate it. Virtually every action we take in our lives begins with a thought, unless we have an instant, subconscious response to a crisis, like jumping out of the way of a speeding car that appears from nowhere while we're crossing the street.

Just as we are what we eat, we are what we think and then what we choose to do as a result of our thoughts. Even the food choices we make begin with a thought. This is why Raja Yoga, the system outlined by Patanjali in the Yoga Sutras, which informs much of the teachings of Deep Yoga, begins by saying that Yoga involves managing the thought waves of the mind. When we allow our thoughts to run wild and expose ourselves to a constant din of commercial messages from mass media, we surrender our destiny into the hands of others whose primary interests are self-serving. When we manage our minds, we become the masters of our destiny.

Thousands of years ago, the Yogis realized that managing their busy minds was a challenge. Imagine that. Long before radio, television, the Internet, video games, Facebook, and text messaging, people found it a challenge to manage their minds. Just think how much more challenging it is today in our fast-paced and over-stimulated world. All the practices of Yoga are designed to support one goal: assisting us in being able to sit still comfortably and relax our minds so that we can come more fully into the present moment and make a connection with our Souls. They key to this is creating a daily practice in our lives, because when we repeat a positive behavior on a consistent basis we unlock the power of ritual.

Since the dawning of civilization, ritual has been at the center of spiritual and cultural practices. We have created ceremonies honoring the rising of the sun, the changing of the seasons, the planting and harvesting of our crops, and the arrival of the new year. These rituals bring us together, lend a deeper meaning to our endeavors, and remind us of our connection with something much larger than our individual selves.

The inherent power of ritual also lies in the fact that repeated activities create patterns in our lives. These patterns then become habits deeply ingrained in our subconscious. Even the simplest of daily rituals can have great benefits. Brushing our teeth gives us the gift of fewer cavities, healthier gums, and fresher breath. Patterning ourselves to get up early gets us to work on time. Keeping things in their proper place makes them easier to find when we need them. On a deeper level, if we sustain a daily ritual of cultivating inner peace, it's more likely that peace will become our nature and habituated way of seeing and dealing with the inevitable challenges of life. If we continuously look to a higher power, we are less likely to get mired in our smaller and self-centered concerns and challenges.

However, the power of ritual can cut both ways. If we anchor deeply into a positive emotion, the whole universe rises up to support us. Likewise, if we anchor deeply into a negative emotion, the whole universe rises up to support us. The tormented soul who turns to drugs and alcohol as their daily ritual faces addiction, depression, and ruin. Constant negative thinking, anger, fear, and indecision, create their own emotional habituations and destructive forces. In essence, we become what we think and what we do, positively or negatively. If we have patterned ourselves through years of repeated negative rituals, changing our ways and healing ourselves can be a daunting task.

Changing the Grooves

Millions of Americans attend Alcoholics Anonymous in hopes of ridding themselves of their drinking problems. It's a thorough and proven program, yet more than ninety percent of people in AA wind up drinking again. This high rate of recidivism also characterizes programs for drug abuse, tobacco addiction, obesity, gambling, and most other personal problems that have become epidemic in modern society. Even if our situation is not extreme and we simply long for personal growth, greater awareness, and deeper meaning in our lives, these aspirations can seem as elusive as it is for the addict seeking recovery. Just witness how often we make simple resolutions for the new year only to find ourselves failing again as we slip back into our old ways.

Among the primary reasons that change is so difficult is that ritualized habit patterns, whether positive or negative, create grooves, known as *samskaras*, in our subconscious mind, which Yoga calls the *chitta*. Chitta can be compared to the hard-drive on our computer. Our daily activities and experiences are the programming stored on the hard-drive. When we resolve to change our behavior, we typically do so with our conscious mind, called manas. If the message from manas fails to permeate down into chitta at the subconscious layer, we don't change those grooves. This sets the stage for failure and causes a dissonance in our psyche that often leads us into even deeper negative behaviors.

A second powerful reason is that our conventional system of treating mental and physical disorders is primarily palliative and disempowering. We are given medications to tranquilize us and mask our depression even though it often arises from our continued over-indulgences. We have pills and potions to ease our pain, curb our appetite, mask our dyspepsia, and counter our sexual dysfunction. Rarely do western doctors prescribe significant and sustained changes in the lifestyles and behaviors that have created or contributed to these maladies. This system is disempowering in that we are led to believe only the experts can treat us, and that we are incapable of taking charge of our own lives and implementing positive changes.

Yoga teaches us that the opposite is true, that we all possess a miraculous inner power to heal and transform our lives. It offers us a host of potent tools to assist our journey. The simple practice of a daily asana, pranayama, and meditation routine begins to lead us towards physical and emotional healing. Practices such as pratyahara (withdrawal of the senses) and pratipaksha bhavana (the cultivation of positive emotions), both of which have been discussed in previous chapters, help deepen our healing and personal growth.

Much of the New Age self-help movement arises from these ancient practices, yet it is often packaged as another quick fix that takes little or no effort. These modern gurus often preach that if you simply visualize that great new job, relationship, or possession that you want so badly, it will be yours in no time at all. The visualization part is largely true. As I said earlier, the whole universe rises up to support our thoughts, positive or negative, and we do tend to manifest what we desire, for better or worse. The missing element in New Ageism is *tapas*, the sustained dedication, self-discipline, and devotion that all the great yogic texts insist is essential to achieving our goals.

The Yoga Sutras of Patanjali hold that self-discipline and devoted practice are essential for transformation and self-realization.

Sutra I:11 *Abhyasa vairagyabhyam tannirodhah.*
The mental modifications are restrained by practice and non-attachment.

The key here is sustained practice, *abhyasa*, and detachment, *vairagya*. When we detach from the constant sensory stimulation in our lives, from our busy minds, and from worrying about the outcome of our efforts, we enter more fully into the present moment.

We stick with our chosen rituals because we understand they are beneficial and transformative even if the results we hope for do not manifest as quickly as we desire. True transformation unfolds organically over time. The idea of a quick fix, which is the promise of most mass media marketing and medications designed to quickly mask our symptoms, is an illusion.

> **Sutra I:14 *Sa tu dirgha kala nairantarya satkarasevito drdhabhumih.***
> Practice becomes firmly grounded when well attended to for a long time, without break, and in all earnestness.

The more we repeat our practice with deep faith and daily devotion, the more it becomes our nature. The more it becomes our nature, the greater our healing and personal growth will surely be. This is *sadhana*, the yogic word for daily practice. If you want Yoga to work its magic for you, establish a sadhana, a practice that nourishes you every day. Tapas is like creating an inner fire to burn away your impurities and help you recreate yourself as more balanced and whole beings. It is an alchemical process that slowly and organically transforms you in body and mind while bringing you into closer touch with Spirit.

Creating and sustained a daily practice, as we all know from new year resolutions that we didn't stick with, is challenging. There is an inner stubbornness within most of us that resists change despite our greatest intentions. So it's always better to seek small victories rather than take on large changes that inevitably doom us to failure. Try a five-minute practice every morning in which you center yourself, breathe deeply, set your intention for the day, and do just a few Yoga poses. Once this is firmly established, you can then lengthen your practice a little, moving slowly forward on a consistent basis.

Below is an example of a very simple and short daily practice. If you are unfamiliar with these basic poses, go online and a simple search will provide you with photographs and basic instructions. During your practice, seek to find the "edge" that is often beyond your comfort range, but never force your body further than it is ready to go. Greater flexibility, balance, and strength come through dedicated practice over time.

A Simple Daily Practice

Posture	Details and Length
Centering Yourself	Begin in a comfortable cross-legged seated posture
8 Steps Into Yoga	Guide yourself through Eight Steps Into Yoga (Chapter 24)
Seated Twist	Hold for five deep breaths on each side
Lateral Extension	Hold for five deep breaths on each side
Forward Fold	Legs straight out, reach for toes—five breaths
Knees to Chest	Laying on back, hug knees to chest for five breaths
Relaxation	Laying on back, straighten legs out on floor for twenty breaths

Again, this is a very simple and short daily practice. If you are well versed in Yoga postures, add or subtract any asanas you like. The main thing is to have a daily practice, a sadhana, that you fully commit to and do every day. It's always best to do your practice first thing in the morning before you begin to address your obligations for the day, because if you put it off until later you greatly diminish the likelihood that you will follow through and do it. This is also why a short practice is advised at the beginning. If you take on too much you are likely to fall off before the ritual has the chance to take hold. Finally, even though these are very simple and therapeutic Yoga poses, never do anything that causes you pain. If you have any medical conditions, consult a Yoga or Ayurvedic practitioner before deciding on what's right for you.

Ancient Wisdom for Modern Times

The Hatha Yoga Pradipika, which was written in the fifteenth century, remains one of the most important texts on Hatha Yoga and echoes the Yoga Sutras on the importance of choosing your life experiences and staying devoted to daily practice:

> I:15 Overeating, exertion, talkativeness, adhering to rules, being in the company of common people, and an unsteady mind are the six causes that destroy Yoga.

> I:16 Enthusiasm, perseverance, discrimination, unshakeable faith, courage, and avoiding the company of common people are the six causes of success in Yoga.

Verse fifteen warns us that allowing our senses to control our lives leads to negative habitual behaviors and poor decisions. By advising that we not adhere to rules, the Pradipika means that the social conventions of society often keep us in a bubble of illusion from which we should extract ourselves. The warning about being in the company of "common people" is telling us that we become like those with whom we associate. The more we spend time with others who blindly follow their senses and are driven by negative habituations, the more we will remain in this state of consciousness as well.

In Verse sixteen the Pradipika reaffirms the need for *tapas*— the practice of persevering at all costs to achieve our goals. This is where the power of positive ritual comes in. The more we take the wisdom of Yoga and apply it to our lives in a pragmatic and consistent way, the greater our personal growth will be. Creating and sustaining new rituals is the key to vanquishing old patterns that inhibit or harm us. This is truly the work of self-transformation. We change our lives by changing our lives, by implementing new behaviors that we know are in our best interest, and repeating them consistently until they become our dominant modes of behavior.

Creating New Rituals

Here are four suggested ways that you can begin to establish new rituals in your life and begin tapping into your own inner power:

- Awaken 30 minutes earlier each morning and take private, sacred time for yourself. Do a few gentle Yoga poses, take some deep breaths, affirm your commitment to personal growth, and see your day as a glorious journey about to unfold (see the chart earlier in this chapter for a simple beginning to a daily practice).
- During your day, avoid negative speech, profanity, and gossip. Engage in more mindful communication. Be positive, compassionate, authentic, truthful, respectful, authentic, and considerate. Contemplate the associations you have in your life that do not serve you well. Resolve to minimize your contact with these people without being hurtful.
- See your body as the temple of your Spirit, and every time you feel drawn towards some behavior that might not be in your best interest, ask yourself if this behavior honors the person you deeply desire to be. Heed the answer that arises from your heart.

- Identify a negative habit that you would like to release. Create a resolve, a *samkalpa*, that states in present tense that you have already achieved your goal. For instance: *My diet is wholesome and pure, and I only eat what I need to nourish myself.* Repeat this resolve over and over to yourself, especially during times of silence and contemplation.

Through embracing simple rituals such as these, you sow the seeds of change in your life. As you sustain these practices over time with dedication and faith, you begin tapping into your inherent inner power. This power is the catalyst that transforms those seeds into sprouts, sprouts into blossoms, and ultimately brings forth the fruits of healing and personal growth. As a result, you will have become the master of your own destiny. This is the true journey into Yoga.

◆ ◆ ◆ ◆ ◆ ◆ ◆ ◆ ◆ ◆

ANCIENT WISDOM
FOR
MODERN TIMES

Moksha

Moksha is liberation.

Knock down all the walls.
Untie all the knots.

Let go of old agreements about who you are.

Embrace your freedom relentlessly.

Sing your unique song of life
each and every day.

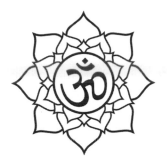

Chapter 24

Your Inner Child

Imagine you're walking down the street with your son or daughter, and you say, "Christmas is coming in just two weeks!"

You think this might give them a thrill of anticipation and be a good topic for a little conversation, but they are likely to answer, "Look at that pretty kitty-cat over there!"

They are more connected. More in the present moment. Seeing the simple miracles all around them. It's only through the socialization process that they learn to get caught up in the past and future, to anticipate better times to come rather than seeing the wonder in their immediate experience. As they get older, they'll learn to long for Christmas and other special events, and they will also learn to fear the future as well, and to hold onto the hurts of their past.

Go to the beach with your child and it's likely that they'll frolic with glee in ocean water you find too cold to keep a toe in for more than a breath or two. They do better with the heat as well. They have more range, a greater capacity to accept—and even revel in—whatever is going on. They have yet to learn to covet all the comforts we become attached to along the way. They can fall down, skin their knees, scream in pain, then jump up and get right back in the game.

We gain much experience and wisdom as we age, which is essential to meet the responsibilities of adulthood, but we lose our inner child along the way. We become increasingly estranged from the present moment. We fixate on the skinned knees. We miss the miracles. When Christmas arrives, we're likely to be saying, "Springtime is just around the corner," while the child answers, "look at the beautiful lights on the tree!"

We also put ourselves in lots of boxes. Smaller and smaller boxes. We lose our openness. We lose our wonder. We lose our innocence, our trust, our hope, our faith. We start to sweat the small stuff. We protect and defend our boxes. We get agitated by experiences outside of the walls we have constructed around ourselves, resistant to change, and set in our ways. We form strong opinions and seek out those who believe as we do, often feeling that those who don't agree with us are our adversaries. We hold onto our hurts. We worry. We suffer. Each of us really needs to find our inner child again and let that child play with reckless abandon.

Your Inner Child is always there, conspiring with your Soul, praying that you will wake up and rejoin the dance of life.

The Ball and Chain

As many of us move through adulthood, we become wanderers in an emotional desert. Imagine, there we are, moving through the dunes of a vast and arid wasteland, a big ball and chain around one ankle. It's terribly hot, and we have hold of that chain, dragging that heavy, black, cast iron ball through the sand. We've even forgotten where we're going. All we're doing is pulling that heavy ball around and bemoaning our plight.

Along comes a desert wanderer who says, "Why are you dragging that heavy thing all over the place?"

"Can't you see it's shackled around my ankle?" we respond in angry defense. "Yes, I can see that," the wanderer says calmly, "but it's not locked!"

We glance down. Oh my God! There's no lock on the shackle. We've been dragging this miserable thing through the desert for years, sweating and toiling, and it's never been locked.

"Just reach down and take that thing off," the wanderer beckons with a gentle smile. This makes immeasurable sense, but something stops us in our tracks. We just can't do it. We don't realize it, but in our deepest subconscious, we are attached to our ball and chain.

Our ego defends, "But this *MINE*, I'm not just going to take it off and leave it here. I've carried it all this way. This is what I do. Who do you think you are telling me otherwise?"

"Okay, so be it," our wanderer replies, "good luck...and goodbye!"

Off he goes, much like the old sage at the Rainbow Waterfall. Of course, the wanderer IS the same old sage. He is our Deeper Voice, our Inner Child, the whisper of our Soul. But we don't listen. We dismiss the old fool. Others gather around us with their balls and chains and we mock the wanderer together. Some of us even suggest he needs a good thrashing. Better for him that he disappeared. If he returns, we'll show him what for!

Some of us, however, just like those who climbed the cliffs to the Rainbow Waterfall, begin to ponder what the wanderer said. We keep dragging our ball and chain for a while, but it's not the same. Finally, we decide to take it off. We're scared to death. What will we do then? Where will we go? What will happen? We feel great resistance and uncertainty. Yet we begin to face the fact that our life is no fun the way it is. We're tired and worn out from being shackled and constrained.

We kneel down...take a deep breath...grasp the shackle and pull it open...lift it off our ankle and drop it in the hot sand.

We slowly stand up...noticing that it suddenly feels cooler...wonderfully cooler.

Our body feels lighter...more supple.

An energy we haven't felt for years runs through us...tingling.

On the horizon...for the first time we can remember...we see some palm trees.

We walk there...it feels like floating without our ball and chain.

It's a magnificent oasis.

We sit by the water...we've never felt better.

We cup a sip in our hands and quench our thirst.

Our parched throat softens.

Something takes us over...we haven't felt it in years...we are smiling!

We stand up again and intuitively start to move our bodies...reveling in our newfound freedom and joy...dancing with glee!

We can't resist...we slip into the water...splash around...utterly immersed in joy!

What were we thinking all this time?

Why didn't we do this years ago?

No matter. We've done it...finally, we've done it!

Releasing Excess Baggage

The ball and chain, as you've already figured out, is all our psychological and emotional baggage. If we eat rotten food, we are going to eliminate it one way or another, yet we tend to ingest bad experiences and impressions and hold onto them as if they were treasures. We drag them around everywhere with us and become so attached that we forget that it's even possible to release them. We spend a fortune on analysts, take antidepressant and sleep medications, tell anyone who will listen how tough life is for us, we even listen to TV and radio talk shows with hosts who make a fortune from complaining and sowing the seeds of anger and discontent. We become so identified with our troubles that our ball and chain becomes our identity and we are scared to death of letting it go!

This is one of the biggest shifts of all:

Contentment is elusive as long as you cling to a false identity.

Your false identity is wrapped up in your perceived hurts, your dramas, your opinions and your judgments.

There's no ball and chain, no lock and key. It's an illusion. You can let it all go.

As true as this is, and as simple as it sounds, it isn't so easy and it takes time and effort. Somehow, when we're not paying attention, that ball and chain finds its way back onto our ankle. We have to kneel down and release it again and again. We must nurture our inner child every day, jump out of our boxes, expand our range, dive into the frigid ocean, dance in the rain, jump in all the puddles. It's a lifetime practice. It's worth it. Give it a try.

Unlocking the Shackles

Sit down in a quiet space and contemplate your ball and chain. What are you holding onto? What hurts, umbrages, past traumas, and negative experiences are you holding onto? What boxes have you stuffed yourself into? How have you constricted your range? Do you have negative judgments and opinions to which you are deeply attached? Do you feel stuck?

Now, journal what came up for you. Make a list. Next, order this list in terms of intensity. Place the smallest stuff at the top of the list, and the deeper, heavier, more intense stuff at the bottom. That's the stuff that is harder to deal with. Don't take it on at first. It's harder to let it go. Look at the top five least intense items at the top of your list. Pick the one you think you can deal with most quickly and easily. See it as a little ball and chain. Visualize yourself reaching down and releasing it, then float-walking through your desert to the oasis and diving into its refreshing waters.

Remember that even this little ball and chain will sneak right back and wrap itself around your ankle when you least expect it. Don't allow this to frustrate you (frustration just creates another ball and chain). Release it repeatedly until it's finally gone. Then you can go onto something else on your list. As you stay with this practice, you'll find that, in time, many of the things on your list simply disappear of their own accord...you don't even have to focus on them. At some point, you'll be ready for the bigger stuff. Don't rush it. Listen to your Inner Child—that aspect of you who will know just the right time.

❖ ❖ ❖ ❖ ❖ ❖ ❖ ❖ ❖ ❖

ANCIENT WISDOM
FOR
MODERN TIMES

OM Tat Sat (I Am That)

Whoever you are,
and wherever you go,
on any continent,
in any country,
you are indigenous.

You are never out of place.
You always belong.
For you are always home,
when you dwell in the heart.

Chapter 25

Eight Steps Into Yoga

Before enlightenment chop wood, carry water.
After enlightenment chop wood, carry water.
Zen Proverb

For centuries in mountainous Asian villages, chopping wood and carrying water were centerpieces of life. Each day, one would trudge down a steep path to the stream, fill two large, wooden buckets with water, attach them to a pole that balanced on their shoulders, and then carry the heavy burden back home. The water cooked their food, bathed their bodies, and cleaned their clothing. Then came obtaining the firewood needed to heat the home, cook the food, and boil the water. It had to be chopped, carried, and stacked. The work was tedious and monotonous, yet an essential ritual of survival.

In our modern lives, we're beset with a host of tedious tasks that might not take as much physical exertion as chopping wood and carrying water, but take much more mental energy and tend to wear us down. Add the pressures of the workplace, the relentless pace of our lives, and the overstimulation of our senses, and it often feels as if things are spinning out of control. We become stressed and depressed, dissatisfied and despondent. We want the world to change so that our discomfort is eased, but this will never happen. Life will always be filled ups and downs, tedium, and banality. Enlightenment is when we realize this. Transformation is when we choose to accept, embrace, and enjoy it.

We are all chopping wood and carrying water in our own way. Sometimes it gets heavy, tedious, and tiring. Sometimes a huge chunk of wood falls on our big toe. Water spills over our shoulders. We get a splinter. We fall down and twist our ankle or get stuck in the mud. We also get great pleasure when we light a fire from all that wood we've carried, warm ourselves by its flames and cook our meal. We find pleasure in drinking the fresh water and bathing ourselves in it. In other words, life is challenging and it's also enjoyable and rewarding.

Before enlightenment, we fixate on getting our pleasures and we bemoan our challenges. After enlightenment, we accept the whole deal. We act skillfully, trying not to drop the wood or spill the water, yet when we do, we don't despair. We figure out how to best clean up the mess, lick our wounds, and get on with it. We enjoy the warm fire to the hilt, but we know there's more wood to chop in the cold morning and we are okay with that, too. Reality is the same as it always was. *We* are different. It's always an inside job. Always. This is the trick.

Moving Beyond the Mundane

When we speak of transformation through Yoga, it's not transforming the world around us, it's the process of transforming ourselves. Yoga is journey of understanding who you truly are at the deepest level, of fully living in the present moment, and of experiencing your relationship with all that is. It is a unification of body, mind, and spirit that connects you to your inner wisdom, which is far more vast and deep than most of us ever imagine.

Great sages have achieved enlightenment through the science of Yoga. The works of luminaries such as Albert Einstein, Joseph Campbell, and Henry David Thoreau are infused with the science and philosophy of Yoga. The tools and techniques of Yoga have helped professional athletes, leaders of industry, stage performers, scientists, artists, and a host of others from all walks of life achieve peak performance in their endeavors.

We might not refine the theory of relativity, further the mythic and archetypal principles of the hero's journey, write the next Walden Pond, or win the New York Marathon, but through merging with our deeper selves, accessing our inner wisdom, and living more fully in the present moment, we experience profound healing, reduced stress, feel more contentment, and move towards manifesting whatever our fullest potential might be. This takes us beyond accepting our lot of chopping wood and carrying water for eternity. It opens the possibility of positive change and full expression of who we are at the most authentic level. In other words, we move beyond the Zen proverb, because once we come to terms with reality, accepting and embracing all that is, new possibilities arise in our lives.

Awareness and Presence

While the science of Yoga is rich and complex, and there are a multitude of practices for body, mind, and Spirit, the underlying theme of all techniques rests upon awareness. Awareness means being fully in the present moment, deeply connected to whatever is transpiring in our lives rather than dwelling in a state of mental wandering into the past and future. In a distracted state, we are disconnected from our inner wisdom, our bodies, and our breath. We are unaware of most of what is happening in the moment because our minds are elsewhere. This inevitably causes us to feel disconnected, anxious, and stressed, and—as we have discussed—creates an inner chemistry of agitation and edginess.

In a state of pure awareness, we are present to everything. This is when wisdom reveals itself. The wisdom within us is more readily accessible, and the intelligence of all that is around us comes forth in myriad ways that are often awe-inspiring. For instance, if you walk past a blooming flower with a distracted mind, you might not notice it at all, or perhaps your mind will register it briefly with something like *pretty flower*. An artist or poet gazing at a flower while fully present to all its glory might be inspired to compose a great poem or paint a work of art. A scientist may look so deeply into the flower that he or she realizes new relationships between the flower and its surroundings and a discovery that helps humankind is in the making.

Awareness, attention, and pure presence also bring us into a spiritual state. We are more in touch with the Spirit within us, and the Spirit within all living things. As we contemplate life in the present moment we have epiphanies about ourselves and about the interrelationships of all things. Life then becomes less mundane and more awe inspiring. Our inner chemistry shifts. Anxiousness is replaced with joy. We become more alive, creative, expressive, vibrant, and enthusiastic. We are harmonized in body, mind, and Spirit. We are in a state of Yoga.

The Eight Steps Into Yoga

In our Deep Yoga Mastery of Life programs we have formulated the Eight Steps Into Yoga as a practical yet powerful way to shift ourselves from an excessively externalized, distracted state of mind, to a deeper, more focused inner state of consciousness. In this process, we move away from the ego and the domination of our dramas, fears, and apprehensions, to the wisdom of our deeper selves and the incredible power of presence.

Step 1: Close your eyes and become aware of the interior spaces of your being. Notice how this simple act creates a subtle shift from externalized to internalized awareness. Notice what it feels like to be you inside.

Step 2: Deepen your breath. Visualize the breath starting down in the bottom of your pelvic bowl, then flowing upwards through your ribs and side body, and finally into your chest. Pause, and then follow the breath as it departs, exhaling from the chest down through the side body, all the way to the bottom of the pelvic bowl. Be aware that your breath is a miraculous gift of life. Receive each inhale as an affirmation and empowerment, release every exhale as a deep healing and letting go.

Step 3: Deepen your awareness of your body. Experience it as the temple of your Spirit, a sacred vessel always here to support you. Let the breath go to all the outer edges of your body and flood all the inner space.

Step 4: Connect now with Mother Earth. Feel her supporting you as you sit or stand. Feel the five elements of earth, water, fire, air, and space in every cell of your body. Remember that you are Mother Earth and she is you.

Step 5: Detach from the stream of thoughts in your mind. Support this with the use of a silent mantra such as *I Am*, silently saying "I" on the in-breath and "Am" on the out-breath (if you already have a short mantra that you use in meditation, this can be substituted for *I Am*). Experience the mantra as a Yoga pose for stilling your mind.

Step 6: Bring your consciousness down to the light of your heart. Visualize a light, like a candle flame, right behind your breastbone. See this as the light of your Spirit and source of your inner wisdom. Breathe deeply into this light, feeling more radiant with every breath.

Step 7: Give yourself the gift of just being here, now, in this eternal moment. In your body, in your breath, in connection with Mother Earth, in the light of your heart—here, now, in this eternal moment.

Step 8: Remember that you always have been, and always will be, completely connected, indigenous wherever you go, one with all that is. You are one with all that is.

You might want to record these eight steps and regularly play them back to yourself in moments of stillness, silence, and contemplation. Notice if you feel more present, softer, and peaceful once you've concluded the practice. When you're faced with major decisions in your life, take a moment to go through the eight steps and then ask your deeper self, your Spirit, for guidance. When you hear your inner voice, commit yourself to embracing the advice. Through this process you are accessing the greatest guru you will ever know: The real you.

These simple eight steps are designed to guide you into the very essence of Yoga. Remember, as Patanjali noted in the Yoga Sutras, Yoga is bringing the mind into a state of calmness so that we become present and aware enough to connect with the Soul. Yoga postures, the asanas that nourish us in so many ways, are just a part of the process, they're not the end in and of themselves. Asanas help us become purified, stronger, more balanced, and more flexible in body and mind so that we can more readily enter states of pure presence and awareness. Breath work, meditation, mantra, and affirmations also support us on this journey, as do a natural diet and mindful lifestyle.

It is, of course, essential to practice and begin to master the various techniques of Yoga. An advanced asana practice brings healing and promotes self-empowerment. Seeking to still our minds and master our breath helps us relieve stress, deal with negative emotions, and make contact with the deeper aspects of ourselves. If, however, we are only practicing Yoga techniques on our mats, we are unlikely to make the sort of progress that is indicative of true growth and transformation.

Along with the Eight Steps Into Yoga, there are a host of ways to take Yoga off our mats and begin to integrate it into our daily lives.

Here are a few you can begin integrating into your daily life starting right now.

Deep Breathing

Become more deeply connected with your breath throughout your day. Teach yourself to breathe deeply and fully in a three-part yogic breath, filling first your abdomen, then drawing the inhale up into the ribs and side body, finally binging the breath all the way up to your heart center. Exhale from the heart center back down through the ribs and side body, and finally back down to the abdomen. This practice can be done virtually anywhere and any time. You can breathe deeply while working at a desk or taking a walk, while riding in a car or standing in a grocery line. Whenever you find yourself becoming distracted, agitated, or imbalanced, remember your breath. Likewise, when you feel joyful and whole, celebrate your breath.

Become More Intimate with Nature

Make a point of seeing the sunrise and sunset as often as possible. At night, pay more attention to the moon and stars. See this as your personal, sacred time when you honor the rhythms of nature and ponder the grandeur of the cosmos. Commit to regular nature walks or hikes, or simply to becoming more aware and appreciative of the flowers, bushes and trees in your neighborhood or workplace...even if there are just a few.

Authentic Speech and Making Time for Silence

Make your speech more authentic, doing your best to speak from the heart. Avoid gossip and negative conversations. Recognize that the language you choose affects your level of consciousness as well as the consciousness of those who are listening. Along with authentic speech, spend more time in silence. Turn off mass media. Avoid noisy and hectic environments. Listen to peaceful and soothing music. Notice how long it takes for the mind to begin to settle once you remove yourself from the normal hubbub of your daily life.

Mindful Eating

Your body is the temple of your Spirit. Everything you ingest becomes part of your body, mind, and Spirit. Try to eat as fresh and organic as possible, focusing on a whole food, plant-based diet. Never ingest junk food or heavily processed foods. Take time to bless each meal in some silent and simple way. Contemplate the abundance of Mother Nature and all the effort that went into bringing this food to you, from those who planted it, nurtured it, and harvest it, to those who brought it to your market. Have gratitude for the entire process. Then, find one day every month to fast, even if it is just skipping one or two meals.

Material Cleansing

Most of us living in the First World have far too much of everything. We are addicted to consuming and collecting, forever seeking an illusory sense of satisfaction through the acquisition of material items. If you stop reading this book right now and go look in your closet and other storage areas, you'll immediately see proof of this. Find time to go through each storage area and get rid of everything you don't truly need. Don't worry about trying to sell it, just give it away to charity and take a tax write-off if this benefits you. You may find a part of your mind fighting you over several items, giving you some seemingly legitimate rationalization for hanging on to this or that. If this comes up for you, use the "one-year rule." If you haven't used something for more than a year, it's time to let it go.

Serving Others

Ahamkara, or the sense of "I-ness," is one of the primary obstacles to Yoga. Ahamkara, in part, means over-identification with the ego, seeing ourselves as the central character in our world, with everything happening to us, for us, or against us. Yoga invites us to transcend the ego and connect with a deeper awareness, perceiving the oneness of our world. A key to accomplishing this is *seva*. Seva means service; giving ourselves to others without any desire for reward or recognition. We can all find ways to serve, from simple strokes to grand gestures. If you are new to seva, I suggest simple strokes. It might be just cleaning up the Yoga Studio you attend after class by helping to put away blankets and props. Perhaps you might choose to pick up litter when you see it as a gesture of seva towards Mother Earth. You might choose to help a friend in need, or volunteer for a few hours at a charitable organization whose mission you believe in. Even small acts such as these help us open to a larger vision of the world than just focusing on what's in it for us.

Gratitude and Divine Awareness

Recognize yourself as a Divine Being. Seek to have your actions be in alignment with this divinity. Ask yourself, "Is this choice I'm about to make honoring the divine within me?" Along with this, attempt to see the Divine in every experience, from the grandeur of nature to the tedious and mundane aspects of daily life. Recognize that there is a Divine Plan and a Divine Essence permeating all things. Have gratitude for all experiences, all difficulties, and all challenges. In cultivating gratitude and recognizing and surrendering to this sense of higher power, you move most closely towards the essence of Yoga.

I recommend that you begin with one or two practices you feel would be the easiest for you. Once you have integrated these shifts into your life, move on to those practices that seem more challenging. The important thing is to make a commitment to opening your heart to your greater potential, implementing positive change, and seeking to live, rather than just practice, Yoga.

◆ ◆ ◆ ◆ ◆ ◆ ◆ ◆ ◆ ◆

ANCIENT WISDOM
FOR
MODERN TIMES

What If?

What if today
you let go of the need to be right?

What if today
you let go of opinions and judgments?

What if today
you said yes every time you felt
like saying no?

What if today
you saw the best in everyone?

Chapter 26
The Light of Love

Who am I?
This is the eternal question for which there is only one answer.
You are love.

It's all about rhythm and harmony. Everything holds vibration. Everything. Even rocks and wood and metal. For a tangible example of vibration let's consider a stringed instrument. If one of its strings is out of tune, any note or chord a musician plays on it sounds dissonant and annoys everyone within earshot. Bring it back into tune, however, and there is harmony, the music sounds soothing and melodious, the instrument has its integrity again. It's the same thing with an auto engine that's running roughly. All the parts get stressed. Performance is impeded. Its life is shortened.

In many ways, you are like a fine instrument. If you live in an environment filled with harsh sounds and hectic activity, it drains you and wears you down. You are likely to feel depleted, stressed, and out of tune. This condition lowers your immune function and sets the stage for illness. It is a *vibrational*, or *energetic* condition, connected to your *energy body*, which has an innate need for harmony.

What Yoga calls the Divine Being within you is known in the Mind/Body medical community as your energy body. There is a growing field of Energy Medicine that treats patients with vibrational frequencies rather than invasive surgeries and heavy drugs. The theory is that when our energy body is in dissonance, the entire organism suffers. Bring it back into harmony, and the organism has greater opportunity to heal and thrive.

The origin of this new field of Energy Medicine dates back to the late 1700s and Homeopathic Medicine. German physician Samuel Hahnemann viewed disease as a disturbance in the energy body (or life force). He believed that patients could be treated with heavily diluted preparations of substances that cause effects similar to the symptoms of the patients. These substances, Hahnemann contended, contain a vibration that supports the energy body in dealing with the disease. Through a process of experimentation on patients, he created scores of what came to be called homeopathic remedies. While Hahnemann's theories did take hold, and homeopathy has grown through time, it remains controversial and rigorously opposed by the mainstream medical community.

Energy Medicine faces an equally powerful opposition from the establishment. As a result, the development of this noninvasive, low cost system of treatment has been greatly hindered. The pharmaceutical industry, which is deeply entrenched with mainstream medicine, views it as a threat to its massive profits. Research grants are difficult to obtain, which further hinders the progress of Energy Medicine, especially the quest to detect minor disturbances in the Energy Body, which could prove to be effective preventive medicine.

Energy Medicine is a scientific approach that is able to integrate science and spirituality, something that has been left out of the mainstream medical model. As Dr. Richard Gerber, a pioneer in this field, notes, "It's only by viewing the body as a multidimensional energy system that we begin to approach how the Soul manifests through molecular biology. The vibrational practitioner influences the individual's consciousness, helping them gain insight into the factors predisposing toward the creation of their illness, or why the illness crystallized at this time in their life."

Divine Rhythms

From a yogic viewpoint, YOU are the vibrational practitioner. You create the harmony and the dissonance in your life. You have the power to tune your instrument, and the more you seek to keep it tuned, the more your life will naturally fall into alignment, balance, and grace.

> *When you align yourself with the rhythms of the Divine, your energy body becomes healed, whole, and vibrant.*
>
> *When you align yourself with the rhythms of the Divine, your life becomes fluid, balanced, and melodious.*
>
> *When you align yourself with the rhythms of the Divine, you greatly increase your capacity to live in contentment and inner peace.*
>
> *When you align yourself with the rhythms of the Divine, you greatly increase your capacity to manifest your fullest potential.*

It all has to do with rhythm. All life on Mother Earth is dancing to a subtle symphony composed by the Divine and performed throughout the cosmos. All galaxies are spinning through space in an elegant dance. As we spin around our sun, the seasons unfold. The moon moves the tides and even influences the fertility cycles of women. As many sacred texts remind us, there is a time for sowing and a time for reaping, a time for action and a time for contemplation, a time for beginnings and a time for endings.

These sacred rhythms even permeate our daily lives. Different species of flowers open their blossoms at precise times of the day. Honeybees are attuned to these patterns, and they plan their flights accordingly. Some plants and animals perform their parts of the symphony during the daylight, while others make their music at night. This twenty-four hour cycle is called "Circadian Rhythm," and all species of life have their melodies and harmonies embedded deeply within their DNA.

When we disconnect from our natural rhythm, we suffer. Our minds and bodies are affected by this dissonance in myriad ways. Jet lag, staying up all night to cram for a test, partying into the early morning hours, and sleeping during the day all have deleterious effects. Much of our modern, artificial society disconnects us from our natural rhythms and promotes physical and mental distress. Healing begins when we reconnect with the Divine and retune ourselves, so that we are again a natural part of the cosmic symphony.

Beyond your body, beyond your mind, you are essentially an Energy Being. This is your Spirit, the Divine Being within you. All energy is a source of power. All energy is a form of fire; it creates heat and light. This is why the journey into awareness is called en*light*enment. We are connecting with our inner light, and we are creating more light—expanding our life force, becoming more radiant.

The home of this Divine Being within you is your heart center. It resides in the center of your chest, just to the right of the organ of your heart. It is often visualized as a golden candle flame just behind the breastbone. This light glows throughout your physical being and gently surrounds you. This surrounding, invisible yet often tangible luminescence is what is referred to as your aura. The more you cultivate your inner light, the more radiant your aura. The more *enlightened* you become. Even if you don't subscribe to the notion of auras, think about those people in whose presence you instantly feel warm and happy, and those in whose presence you feel uncomfortable and distant. You are feeling into their energy bodies.

This light is at the heart center, this inner vibration, when connected to Spirit, is the vibration and light of love.

Love is the underlying energy that governs all that is throughout the cosmos.

Love is the greatest healing force in the world.

Love is always, at every turn and in every way, the ultimate answer.

Unfolding the love inherent within you is the path to spiritual transformation.

You are the embodiment of the Light of Love.

What the science of Energy Medicine is just beginning to discover saints and sages have known it throughout the ages. It's not romantic love, with all its illusions and misunderstandings. It's Universal Love. The Cosmic Rhythm. The Song of the Divine. The Source of All That Is.

We have a choice. Our lives can be discordant, fraught with sharp and strident notes, riddled with nonsensical and contradictory lyrics, out of tune and painful to endure. Or, we can create a harmony that resonates within us and with the world around us. The song of our life can be filled with doubt, anger, fear, judgment, hate, anxiety and malaise, or it can be a masterpiece of contentment, compassion, gratitude, acceptance, peace, and loving kindness.

One song is a ballad from Hell, the other is a symphony from Heaven. It's your choice. Which do you choose?

◆ ◆ ◆ ◆ ◆ ◆ ◆ ◆ ◆ ◆

ANCIENT WISDOM
FOR
MODERN TIMES

The Pancha Mahabhutas

*The mahabhutas are the five elements
that comprise all that is.*

Earth.

Water.

Fire.

Air.

Space.

Feel them in every cell of your body.

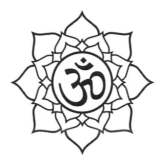

Chapter 27

Aligning with the Divine

Have you ever been in a balance pose, standing there on one leg with a dozen other Yoga students in class, and suddenly you realize that you are about to lose it? Your muscles tense, your hips sway back and forth, the sole of your standing foot arches and flexes, and squirms, your arms flail in the air...and then you do lose it and have to bring the raised leg down to the mat or fall over and crash to the floor. It's often a little embarrassing and frustrating, you might even feel agitated and angry with yourself, but you know it's a sign that you are out of alignment and need to practice that pose more regularly until you have it mastered.

This experience is a great physical metaphor for being aligned, or not aligned, with the Divine. The Divine can also be called dharma, which means Universal Law. These are the principles that govern everything in the universe and the cosmos beyond. When NASA scientists have everything in alignment with cosmic laws they can land a rocket on Mars. If not, the rocket crashes or becomes lost in space. When we are aligned with the laws of gravity, we can hold a balance pose. Otherwise, we fall. When we are aligned in body, mind, and spirit, we experience healing, transformation, and inner peace. Otherwise, we suffer.

Most, if not all of us, come to Yoga because we are suffering. We might have physical aches and pains, mental stress and anxiety, or perhaps a deep inner longing to find more depth and meaning in our lives. Yoga teaches us that all such suffering is a signal that we are out of alignment with our higher self, with dharma and with the Divine, and that this suffering is a calling for us to reevaluate and change our lives. As I noted in the chapter titled Yoga of the Heart, the key to realignment is learning to listen to the inner voice that whispers from our heart center, which is the true seat of our deeper consciousness.

Healing Rhythms

When I was attempting to heal many years ago from stage four cancer and a broken back, I began following a deep inner urge to get up in the dark of early morning and ride my bike to a dock on San Diego Bay where I would meditate to the rising sun. As the sun crested over the rolling hills beyond the bay, I experienced a golden beam of its light streaming directly into my heart center. As this happened I heard the whisper of an inner voice. It was not the usual thought streams of my mind. It was a voice of inner knowing that felt like it came from the center of my chest. As the cynicism of the former journalist inside of me began to scoff at this, I decided to make a shift and heed the wisdom of this inner voice in every way possible. As a result, I found myself at the water's edge almost every morning despite the great physical and mental challenge of sticking with it.

This inner voice also told me that it was imperative to fast for days at a time and to only eat organic vegetarian food. This process, which was also challenging, eventually took eighty pounds off of my body and ultimately became what I called "organic chemotherapy" as I detoxified my body and healed from the cancer. The same voice also guided me into deep breathing and doing Yoga postures on a daily basis, often for several hours per day, on my own and in classes. This led to healing my back as well.

Later, as I studied the great texts of Yoga and Ayurveda, I found many of the practices that my inner voice was guiding me towards were right there in those ancient teachings. This wasn't because I was anyone special or insightful. The reason, I came to understand, is that we all possess this inner knowing. Some of us never connect with it. For others, there are intermittent moments when we tune into what we often call intuition or gut feelings. Most of us have experienced this. I'm sure you can remember many times when you responded to an inner knowing and the result was favorable, and many times when you chose not to follow you inner wisdom and paid a price for it.

I was fortunate enough to have brought myself back from the brink, from profound misalignment and suffering to health and wholeness, through the process of this listening and taking determined and sustained action. Along the way, I realized that no matter how miraculous healing from a broken back, failed surgery, and stage four cancer might seem, this also was not special or unique. We all have an incredible inner power to overcome obstacles, heal to our maximum potential, and move forward in our lives with greater vibrancy and clarity.

The healing process often begins with taking stock of our lives and coming to understand our imbalances and the habits that sustain them. This is where both Ayurveda and Yoga come into play. Both sciences offers us many overlapping tools and techniques, teaching us that the knowledge and the wisdom needed to guide us into greater harmony and balance exist within each one of us. If we learn to listen, that deeper inner voice of our consciousness will always tell us what is right and what is wrong. It will also lead us to our highest aspirations and the fullest potential of self-expression in our lives. In the individual sense, this defines dharma: finding that path in our lives which is truly what we were meant follow.

Learning to Listen

In the Yoga Sutras, Patanjali gives us what he calls the three sources of pramana, which means right knowledge of that which was previously unknown. The first and most important is pratyaksha, which means having a direct experience of something. We might read or hear about the wonders of love and horrors of war, but until we experience them we will not a full understanding of what they are. The second source is *anumana*, which means inference. For instance, if we see smoke rising above the horizon we can reasonably infer there is a fire of some sort that caused it. The third source is called *agama*, which is the written or spoken testimony from those who have become self-realized. Buddha, Christ, and Patanjali would fall into this category, as would all the major scriptures that have held true throughout the ages.

Because we are Divine Beings and the wisdom of all humankind is encoded within us, our inner voice is speaking from an inherited memory of direct experience. It is essential, however, not to delude ourselves or allow the ego-mind to trick us into thinking it is the deeper mind. *Viparaya* and *vikalpa*, Patanjali says, are the main forms of wrong knowledge, delusion, and false information. Advertising often falls into these categories, promising more than the product can deliver, making specious claims, and seeking to lure us into believing in something that is untrue. We all have an inner sense of things that seem too good to be true, yet we still find ourselves getting drawn in as a result of being excessively focused on our desires.

Even though this voice of the soul is always whispering to us, all too often our minds are so distracted and busy that we just don't hear. Still, when we engage in an activity that is out of alignment, such as overeating, drinking too much alcohol, using drugs, telling little white lies, gossiping, or being excessively judgmental, we always know deep inside that we are not acting in our best interest or honoring who we are at the most authentic and conscious level. We can even watch ourselves engaging in this or that unconscious behavior as we feel powerless to resist the compulsion. Haven't we all had this experience?

This phenomenon of acting out of harmony with our innate wisdom creates inner tension and dissonance, leaving us unhappy with ourselves. Who hasn't felt this way as well? Such constant discomfort leads us to seek more distractions, which further feed our bad habits and take us even farther away from our true selves. It is a spiral into darkness. Yoga and Ayurveda beckon us back to the light. First, we purify ourselves with organic, natural food. We strengthen and open our bodies through asana poses. We enhance our life-force energy through pranayama. We regain control of the mind and senses through mantra, meditation, and withdrawal from the hectic pace and noise of modern life. We are invited to follow moral precepts and observances that make us more peaceful, honest, self-reliant, and aware of the higher forces of nature.

During this process, we open our hearts more fully and hear the inner whisper of our soul more clearly. We learn, through ritual and repetition, to act on that wisdom and transform our lives to a higher level of awareness and behavior. The result is self-healing, greater clarity, and a sense of contentment that eventually allows us to leave our lives of agitation and distraction behind. Most of us won't master all these practices, and each one takes great time and devotion, but progress is inevitable as long as we apply ourselves with consistency, determination, and devotion.

It is an amazing and transformative journey, but it is also very challenging. Our habits are deeply ingrained and can only be overcome through great courage, faith and discipline, which are called *virya*, *shrada*, and *tapas*. This is true even in the performing of physical postures. If we are having trouble balancing on one leg, we must practice that pose repeatedly. Through this process we teach the muscles and bones the proper alignment to support our body as we teach the mind to shift from fear, doubt, and apprehension about the balance to courage, calmness, and confidence. Through the ritual of repetition, we undergo a transformation, and the pose that was once so frustrating eventually becomes one of self-empowerment and self-expression.

This process is essential for changing any aspects of our lives that we know are not in our best interest. We must find a positive habit and repeat it until it replaces the negative habit and our lower impulses no longer control our behavior. I remember how challenging it was to change my diet and to fast for prolonged periods of time. It was equally challenging to get out of my warm bed before sunrise to begin a day of healing practices. Over time, however, these practices became my nature, and the old behaviors that contributed to the cancer and constant pain that almost ended my life melted away. As a result, I had a direct experience of the capacity we all have for self-healing.

This is the essence of aligning ourselves with the Divine and with the divinity of our own souls, and it is accomplished by altering our behaviors. Ayurveda and Yoga not only offer us the necessary guidance and practices to achieve this alignment, they also lead us to the greatest guru we will ever have in our lives. This guru is our inner self, the voice that is whispering in your heart even as you read these words. It is ever beckoning you to heal and transform, to manifest your highest aspirations, and to dwell eternally in the contentment, wellness, and love that is waiting to blossom within you as you align yourself with the Divine.

Divine Alignment Practice

As a practice, sit in a comfortable cross-legged position. Softly close your eyes and begin to contemplate a major problem or decision with which you have been grappling. Do the work inside your brain and go over all the possible solutions and obstacles that have already come to mind.

After a few minutes of this contemplation, cross your palms over your heart center. Deepen your breath and become aware of a flame, like a golden candle flame, right behind your breastbone. See this as the light of your Soul, the fountain of your inner wisdom, your inner guru. Very gently now, present your question or problem to your heart. Be silent and still. Breathe deeply, slowly, and smoothly. Be patient. Your answer, your inner knowing, should arise within just a few minutes. If you don't hear your inner voice on the first attempt, it's likely that the outer mind is still too turbulent. This is common, so don't be discouraged. Repeat the practice over the next several days until the answer comes, as it eventually will. When you receive the answer, embrace it with courage, faith, and self-discipline.

Please don't wait to do this. The essence of Yoga is not reading, studying, or knowing, it is in the doing. There's no better time to begin your journey into aligning with the Divine than with your very next breath.

◆ ◆ ◆ ◆ ◆ ◆ ◆ ◆ ◆ ◆

ANCIENT WISDOM
FOR
MODERN TIMES

Knowledge versus Wisdom

*Knowledge
is essential for our
personal growth.*

*Wisdom is putting that
knowledge
into action.*

*Knowledge without action
is like a seed without water,
unable to fulfill its potential beauty.*

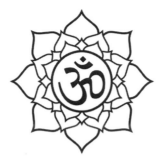

Chapter 28
The Guru Is You

I was walking through a peaceful forest of oak and pine in the mountains of Idyllwild during our annual Mastery of Life Retreat at the Zen Mountain Center, a Buddhist Monastery on three hundred twenty-five acres of wilderness just below the Pacific Crest Trail. It was a typically warm Southern California fall day, and I had wandered into the woods, as I often do during a break, to drink in the healing grace of nature. There was a gentle breeze whispering through the air. The vibrant blue sky was framing stone mountaintops rising above the timberline, with an occasional thick, white cloud perched on a peak like an angel's pillow.

Just before the break, I had been talking to our Deep Yoga students about the incredible power of growth and transformation that each one of us possesses. This is a recurring theme in our teachings, yet it is always a challenge to communicate the depth of this truth. Our culture has disenfranchised us from this inner power. We are taught, systematically, that this power is rare...that it resides in the hands of those our media celebrates for their economic, scientific, artistic, or athletic achievements, but never in the grasp of we lesser mortals.

They are the superstars. We are the mundane masses. We can only watch with awe as others achieve greatness. We must seek our power externally, relying upon "experts" to guide and heal us. As a result of our presumed mediocrity we are often hesitant to take responsibility for our actions, our bodies, our minds, or our lives for fear we might fail if we do. So we surrender to the system and look to it to cure our ills. If we eat pepperoni pizza all day and end up with an acid stomach, all we need is a prescription for a purple pill. If our minds are in a constant whirl and we feel anxious and stressed, there are professionals willing to listen to us complain—for a hefty fee, of course—and then put us on antidepressants. If we feel spiritually lost, organized religion or a spiritual master can intercede with the Divine on our behalf.

So it is always important to convey to every student just how amazingly gifted and powerful they truly are. They have heard it so many times before, as children being told by their parents that they can grow up to be anything they choose, and from motivational gurus who urge them to take charge of their lives and step up to their greatness—through a special program that costs several thousand dollars of course. Yet for most it just seems too good to be true, something that happens for other people, but not for them.

I was strolling under a great oak tree as I pondered this on my walk in the woods when I felt something crunch beneath my foot. As I gazed toward the forest floor, I saw that I was surrounded by acorns. Kneeling down, I took one in my hand and noticed how beautiful it was. The little amber, conical seed smoothly flowed out from under a crusty brown cap that looked a little like a French beret. There were hundreds of acorns lying in the pine needles around me, like a village of tiny infants waiting for their moment to sprout and grow. While I'm far from the first person to contemplate the wonder of a mighty oak rising from such a tiny seed, it struck me in a deep, experiential way, as if the acorn and the oak tree from which it fell were offering me a teaching.

I looked up at the thick branches of the great oak twisting into the morning sky, as if reaching up and touching fingers with the Divine. I could feel its massive roots penetrating the earth below me. The prana, or primal life force of the oak tree, was palpable, like a magnetic field surrounding me. I could feel the pure potential of the acorn in the palm of my hand, as if it was whispering, "I am that mighty tree towering above you."

I realized on a deeper level than ever before that the single acorn in my palm contained within it an endless number of oak trees and acorns going back through all time to the first acorn and forward into the future as well. It contained the pure intelligence of this particular life form, all the wisdom needed to grow into a glorious tree and create thousands more acorns; each with the same amazing potential to become mighty oaks and create more acorns.

Of course, many of the acorns around me would simply end up in the bellies of the squirrels I noticed skittering in the trees and bushes around me, or they would be consumed by deer or the birds whose songs are part of the natural music of the Zen Center. Even then, the tiny seed within each nut might find its way from a belly to fertile soil and an opportunity to sprout. Other acorns would simply decompose and return to Mother Earth, but the potential was there in every one of them, just as it is within every one of us.

I gathered up several dozen acorns and headed back to the Zendo before our students returned, placing a single acorn at the foot of each Yoga mat. When we resumed our program, I invited our students to pick up their acorns and examine them. I then asked, "How many oak trees are in the acorn you are holding?"

Most chose "one tree" as their answer, which is logical at first blush. I encouraged them to go deeper in their contemplation, and consider how many acorns as well as trees might be in each acorn. After some silence there was a collective dawning as several whispered at once, "It's endless." They had it! The pure potential of every acorn is infinite.

The next step was obvious to all. "How many human beings, how much human intelligence and power is within each of you?" An answer wasn't even necessary. The tiny acorns had provided the teaching and illustrated the point with grace. Each of us has a profound capacity, given us at birth, to create, manifest, and achieve at a level far higher than most of us are willing to embrace. At the very core of our being lies a timeless wisdom; an innate knowing that is both primal and cosmic.

This is what the ancient sages of Yoga tapped into as they meditated in their Himalayan caves. By looking within to the very core of their beings, they accessed the "seed wisdom" of life. From this Divine Insight, they composed the Vedas, the ancient spiritual texts from which Yoga and Ayurveda arise. These sacred sciences are like fruit from the spiritual tree of the Vedas that provide a method for applying this divinely revealed wisdom to our lives.

If acorns had a human level of consciousness, they too would be able to look deeply within their core and unlock the secrets of the seed within them. But of all life here on Earth only we are blessed with this ability, and it did not begin or end with sages of bygone times. Few of us have the time, discipline, or devotion to unlock all that lies within us. The few who do accomplish this become our saints and sages.

While we are not likely to become Buddha or Christ in this lifetime, we all have experienced those wondrous moments when our confusion dissolves and a higher truth unfolds. We all have heard a deeper voice within us urging us to change course and align our lives with something far greater than our base instincts and mundane desires. When we have chosen to honor this voice, things have usually worked out for the better because we are accessing something profoundly powerful and sacred, something far greater than our individual existence.

The very essence of this inner wisdom is an energetic power, an atomic light that is at the core of our being. Through accessing this power, we can enhance our lives in myriad ways. We can liberate ourselves from the tyranny of our social conditioning. We can heal, transform, and manifest our very greatest self. We can release our limiting dramas, find inner peace, and discover our true calling in life. We can stretch ourselves far beyond our perceived limitations, express ourselves in untold ways, inspire others, and make a contribution to humankind no matter how small or humble it might be.

The Archetypes of Yoga

The wisdom of Yoga and Ayurveda is embedded in numerous texts that came after the Vedas, including the Upanishads, Bhagavad-Gita, Ramayana, and Yoga Sutras of Patanjali. All these ancient works advise us that desire, self-centeredness, greed, and indulgence are pathways to suffering, and that we must transcend the ego to discover who we truly are. Woven into many of these teachings is a great pantheon of deities, including Brahma, Vishnu, Shiva, Krishna, Kali, Durga, Rama, Lakshmi, Hanuman, and Ganesh, just to name a few. For thousands of years, these deities have been carved in wood and stone, depicted in elaborate paintings, and worshipped in temples and at shrines. This has caused many cultures and religions to denounce this spirituality as polytheistic and pagan.

I see a much different picture. These deities are archetypes, embodiments of the forces of life, aspects of the human psyche, symbols of the greatest potential that lies within all of us. Rama, the central character of the Ramayana, personifies the courage, faith, and self-discipline of standing in our truth—our dharma—no matter what obstacles we face. Kali, the Goddess associated with feminine creative power, and *shakti*, the cosmic energy of the Universe, stands for time and change, and symbolically slices our heads off with a sharp knife to destroy our ego. Krishna, the central character of the Bhagavad-Gita, embodies the spiritual power of Divine Love. Shiva, who is mentioned in numerous texts, is the Great Destroyer, the original Yogi, the embodiment of pure consciousness. It is Shiva who visits great suffering upon us, pounds us into the ground and takes everything away, compelling us to shift our perspective, find our inner strength, and transform our lives, or else.

The great adversaries and demons found in many of these ancient texts are also archetypes, like the demon Ravana whom Rama must overcome to rescue his beloved partner, Sita. The armies that Arjuna faces on the battlefield of life in the Bhagavad-Gita are personifications of the multifaceted ego in all its dark manifestations. In these and most all other spiritual stories from the tradition of Yoga it is always a struggle between the good within us and the bad. It is the darkness versus the light. This is the essence of the word *guru*. *Gu* in Sanskrit means dark, *ru* means light. The guru is that which moves us from the darkness to the light, and the greatest guru you will ever meet has been with you since the moment you were born. The guru is you.

Owning Your Power and Living Your Truth

Just as we should never surrender our consciousness to crass materialism or mass marketing, we should never surrender our spiritual quest into the hands of an external guru. Many such gurus are charlatans. Others are secretively obsessed with their powers. The few true gurus in the world never demand nor even ask that you join the flock, pay a tithing, or touch their feet. They merely serve as mirrors so that you might see who you truly are. When you find such a guru, be in their presence often. Give them your attention, your respect, and your devotion. Lay your ego at their feet and allow them to do with it as they choose, but never surrender your inner power. Be the master of your own destiny, ever and always remembering who you really are. You are the acorn with the capacity to manifest a might oak. You are all the archetypes that have ever been, and you have untold powers of self transformation.

The journey of Yoga is a pilgrimage to this inner power. All practices of Yoga are designed to guide you home to truth of who you really are and unfold the potential that has always been within you. When you merge with the inner power you are merging with the Divine, because just as Mother Earth is you and you are her, The Divine is you and you are That. This truth is embodied in the ancient Sanskrit mantras *Aham Brahmasmi*, which means I and the Divine are one, and *OM Tat Sat*, or I am That. You are that which is everlasting and ever knowing.

This is the core teaching of Deep Yoga: The Guru is You. Our dedication is to guiding students towards their fullest potential, encouraging them to bring forth the best in themselves, to own their power and live their truth. We do this with a sense of humility and gratitude, always seeking to align our teachings with the ancient wisdom of Yoga and the Vedas. We are servants as much as we are teachers, and we bow to you, whoever and wherever you are, because we know that You Are That.

◆ ◆ ◆ ◆ ◆ ◆ ◆ ◆ ◆ ◆

Thirty Days of Deep Yoga

Contemplations,

Inspirations

&

Practices

The following practices are excerpted from my Deep Yoga Sacred Practices Blog (www.deepyogablog.com). They are designed for daily inspiration and to facilitate making small yet significant shifts in your life that will open your heart more fully, lead you into greater balance and harmony, and positively alter your view of yourself and the world in which you live.

I recommend you read one per day, meditate on it, and implement the suggested practices in your own unique and intuitive way. Don't try to take on too much or change too many things about yourself all at once. Be gentle and loving with yourself. Anchor in to practices that resonate with you and release those that don't resonate right now.

You might enjoy keeping a brief journal of your experiences so that you can periodically revisit it and remember the most poignant and inspiring experiences that you have on your journey into Deep Yoga.

Day One

Steps

In a moment, softly close your eyes.

Let your awareness flow down from your mind

to your heart center.

Visualize a golden flame of light there.

Anchor into that.

Breathe deeper and fuller.

Feel an inner stillness and silence.

Then ask, "What is a positive step I can take today

that furthers my journey towards fulfilling my Soul's

deepest and most authentic calling."

Listen closely.

The answer will arise with surprising swiftness.

Then, at some point today, take that step.

Day Two

Affirming

Affirm everyone who crosses your path today.
Make no exceptions.
Affirm those you love, those you like, all colleagues
and acquaintances, even those
with whom you might usually disagree.
It needn't be spoken.
Hold a sense of inner affirmation
where appropriate.
Vocalize it where you feel it
might be needed.
The most important part of this practice is to
cultivate affirmation within yourself.
Breathe in acceptance and affirmation.
Exhale acceptance and affirmation.

Day Three

Experiment

Experiment today. All day.
Be an alchemist of your inner chemistry.
Simply chant OM Shanti silently with
every breath you take.
OM is the sound of all creation, and
Shanti is Sanskrit for peace.
By silently chanting this simple mantra
you create the neuropeptides of peace
within your body.
You tune your inner rhythms to softness, suppleness,
acceptance, gratitude
and lovingkindness.
Chant OM Shanti all day long.
Notice your inner space.
Be a beacon of peace.

Day Four

Listen

Shhhhhhh....
Stop.
For just two minutes.
Be still.
Listen.
Notice the sounds that are most distant.
No need to identify, analyze or judge them.
Just notice.
Then notice the sounds closer to you.
Just notice.
Finally, notice the subtle sound of your
breath rising and falling.
Just notice.
Shhhhhh.

Day Five

Expand

Expand your range today.
Drive to work by a different route.
Order something different
from the menu when you go out to eat.
Sing out loud as you walk down the street.
Watch the sunset.
Jump in the cold ocean.
Climb a little mountain.
Roll on the grass.
Dig your fingers into the moist earth.
Put on your favorite music and dance with reckless
abandon.
Expand your range today.

Day Six

Exhale

Today. All day.
Focus on your exhale.
Be conscious of making it a little longer
and slower than your inhalation.
Notice what it feels like in your
physical body to let the breath go.
Notice what it feels like in your
emotional body to let the breath go.
If and when little challenges arise, meet and greet
them with a beautiful exhale.
Notice how you feel.
Notice what happens.
Today. All day.
As often as you can remember,
Focus on your exhale.

Day Seven

Go Home

Go home today.
In every breath you take.
In every pause between your thoughts.
In every action.
Go home.
Go home to your heart.
Feel your soul shining inside you like a
radiant candle flame.
Ask what love would do in every situation.
Listen for the whisper of a voice deep within.
Go home today.
In every breath you take.
In every pause between your thoughts.
In every action.
Go home to your heart.

Day Eight

Choose Love

Choose love today.
In every breath.
In every thought.
In every word.
In every deed.
Ask yourself, "What would Love do?"
When challenges come your way,
as they so often do,
Ask yourself, "What would Love do?"
Choose love as often as you can.
Give it to everyone and everything
with reckless abandon.
Choose love today.
Watch what happens when you do.

Day Nine

Darkness to Light

Release yourself
from the darkness
through seeking the light.
Never meet darkness with darkness,
but meet all that you face with
radiance and light.
Through this practice you will surely
find your way,
and one day, perhaps, have the
great privilege
of guiding others towards the light as well.
Release yourself
from the darkness
through seeking the light.

Day Ten

Reveal Yourself

Reveal yourself to the Divine in every moment.
No matter where you are or what you are doing, feel
something sacred surrounding you.
Then feel that same sense of
sacredness within yourself.
See the Divine in every flower and tree,
in the sky and in the breeze,
in all living things.
As you do, feel connected at the level of Spirit.
Know that everything is a miracle,
and that grace permeates our world.
Reveal yourself to the Divine in every moment,
and the Divine
will reveal itself to you.

Day Eleven
A Small Step

Take a small step today.
Move softly in the direction of something
you've been wanting to bring into your life.
There's no need to rush towards it.
Just turn towards it and take small step.
Notice how this subtle shift changes
the horizon line of your life.
Tomorrow, or perhaps the next day,
take another small step.
Move closer. Softly, lovingly.
Breathing into it without expectation or urgency.
Take a small step today.
Move softly in the direction of something you've
been wanting to bring into your life.

Day Twelve

Forgiveness

Today, fully forgive
the person in your life who has most
criticized you and held you back.
The one who has whispered throughout the years
that you aren't smart or strong or worthy enough to
achieve your greatest aspirations.
Give that person you unconditional forgiveness
for all the hurt they have caused you,
all the doubt and low self-esteem.
Let a vision of that person
come into your awareness.
Notice that you are forgiving is yourself.
Go ahead, forgive yourself.
And then go climb your mountain.

Day Thirteen
Hug Yourself

I invite you to lie on your back
and hug your knees into your chest.
As you breathe deeply, visualize that
you are hugging yourself.
Ask your heart what it is you need right now.
Courage or contentment? Power or peace?
Gratitude, forgiveness, acceptance or
lovingkindness?
Whatever arises, offer it to yourself.
At the same time, receive it.
As you do, embrace yourself
fully and completely.
Hug yourself like you have
never hugged before.

Day Fourteen

Your Aspiration

What is your greatest aspiration?
Say it to yourself…right now.
Say it again and again and again.
Go to the mountaintop and shout it out loud.
Stroll the beach and whisper it endlessly.
Remind yourself of it when you awaken.
Let it be the last thing you say
before you go to sleep.
What is your greatest aspiration?
Say it again and again and again.
Because the more you do,
the more you will find the power to move towards it,
until that day when your
beautiful aspiration is fully realized.

Day Fifteen

Surrender

Among the most courageous of acts
Is letting go.
Act as skillfully as you possibly can.
Then surrender the outcome of your actions
To your sense of higher power.
Let go of the need to control,
The fear that things might turn out
differently than you intend.
Do your best.
Stay committed.
Have great faith in yourself.
Then let go.
The power of surrender will
reveal itself to you as soon as you do.

Day Sixteen

Log In

Login today.
Not onto Google or Facebook or Twitter.
Login to the cosmic Internet.
The wifi is the light of your heart.
The password is OM.
Login now.
Just bring your consciousness
into your heart center, visualize the
flame of spirit there,
silently chant OM and connect with the
eternal and Divine.
Then send a message to whole universe.
A message of love, of inclusion, of grace,
of your soul.

Day Seventeen

Request Organic

When you are at the market, or out to eat, request
organic.
Organic farmers have committed themselves to your
health and to honoring Mother Earth.
Factory farm vegetables are filled with pesticides and
herbicides. Runoff from these crops pollutes our
waterways and contribute to a host of diseases,
including cancer.
Seek to honor those who seek to honor us.
Request organic.
Let your grocer and favorite restaurants
know how you feel.
Make the request.
Let yourself be heard.

Day Eighteen
Deep Within You

What is silence
to you?
When you slip more fully
into the present moment,
what is your experience of it?
When you listen to the
whisper of your breath
what does it say to you?
When you visualize the
flame of spirit
at your heart center,
how does that feel?
When you realize that you truly are
one with all that is,
how can you help but smile?

Day Nineteen
Sharing the Flame

Light a candle,
and with that flame
You can light a dozen more candles,
a thousand more candles.
Each of those new candles that you light
can light a dozen more candles,
A thousand more candles.
Through this journey of
Deep Yoga that we are sharing,
You are igniting the flame of your inner wisdom.
At some point in your journey,
When the time is right,
You will light a dozen more candles,
A thousand more candles.
You will help illuminate the world.

Day Twenty

A Clearing

Look through your closets and cupboards,
Find all the stuff you've stashed for years.
Pack it up and give it away.
Not to your friends or loved ones.
Give it to those truly in need,
To charities who serve the
poor and disenfranchised.
Or pack it into your car and drive to
where homeless people live.
There's a place in almost every city these days.
Give them your stuff.
As you do, ask them their names so that
they truly feel seen.
Wish them all the best.
Hold love for them in your heart.

Day Twenty One
Just Say Yes

Imagine embracing all that is.
Being open to receive and accept
whatever comes your way.
Riding the ups and downs of the day
with a soft smile and open heart.
Imagine affirming everyone
with no exceptions.
Seeing the best and them and
seeing the best in yourself.
Imagine saying yes,
and then saying yes again and again.
Imagine being so openhearted today,
that you just say yes to everything
that comes your way.

Day Twenty Two
Be Wild

Be wild all day.
Celebrate your body.
Celebrate your breath.
Feel them dance with one another.
An in-breath expanding the reach.
An exhale guiding the footfall.
Feel rivers of life coursing through you.
Find those same rivers in the sky.
In the veins of every leaf.
In the eyes of all.
Take a few minutes when you are alone,
And dance ecstatically,
Celebrating the awesome miracle of being.
Be wild. Be uninhibited.
Be free.

Day Twenty Three

Surrender

Raise a white flag inside your heart
today and surrender.
Stand your armies down.
Send the corporals and sergeants
home to their families.
Melt your weapons and forge
instruments of song.
Let your anthem be one of inclusion
and acceptance.
March to the tune of
lovingkindness and compassion.
Hold a drumbeat of peace within your soul.
Raise a white flag inside your heart
and surrender.

Day Twenty Four

Guiding Light

Open the door
To the cave of your heart,
And silently slip inside.
Softly approach the altar.
Sit and gaze gently at the golden flame.
Allow it to illuminate you.
Reach out.
Hold the flame in the palms of your hands.
Notice that it warms, but never burns.
With gratitude and humility,
take the flame back into your world.
Whenever anyone feels lost in darkness
and reaches out to you,
Hand them the light
so that they might find their way.

Day Twenty Five
Small Stuff

Let go of the small stuff today.
Most troubles and concerns,
judgments and attitudes,
fears and apprehensions,
are just that...
small stuff.
Let go of the small stuff today,
as many times as you need to.
Then open your arms wide
to the big stuff.
The miracle of being alive.
The joy of having friends.
The endless possibilities
of being you.

Day Twenty Six

New Ways

Find a new way today.
Change a routine...
just because.
Wear something you haven't worn in ages.
Take an alternate route to work.
Eat something different for lunch.
Listen to new music...
and dance to it.
Break out of any boxes
you've secretly been keeping yourself in.
Find a new way today
to do something simple,
something that you've always done
in a certain way.

Day Twenty Seven

Windows

We often sit in the darkness,
praying for light.
All the time, the light is there.
Everywhere and always.
We block it out with our woes.
Then forget the light we long for is there.
Always there.
There are trillions of cells in your body.
Visualize them all.
Imagine a tiny window covers every cell.
Then breathe in deeply,
and as you exhale,
Throw every window wide open
and let the light flood in.

Day Twenty Eight
A Small Step

Take a small step today.
One that's been calling out to you
from the level of the soul.
Make it a small step in a different direction.
Open to what arises as you do this.
How does it feel to be lightly outside of the
boundaries you have created for yourself?
Is it as frightening as you thought, or does it
feel fraught with potential?
Take a small step today.
A step in a different direction.
One that's been calling out to you from
the level of the soul.
Your greatness awaits you.

Day Twenty Nine

The Conversation

Today. All day.
Have a silent conversation.
Listen to the whisper of your breath.
The subtly different song of the
inflow and the outflow.
Let it be a wordless conversation
with the present moment.
Even during busy times, hold the
conversation like a precious gem.
It is a conversation with life.
A conversation with the present moment.
A conversation with Spirit.
Today. All day.
Have a silent conversation.
Listen to the whisper of your breath.
Better yet, do all three.

Day Thirty

The Prayer

Find a moment today, when no one is watching.
Or everyone is watching.
Fall to your knees and kiss the earth.
Thank your sense of higher power for the astonishing
miracle of being you.
Give thanks for the songs of birds,
the morning breeze,
The sunrise and sunset,
The night sky splashed with stars that
speak of distant galaxies.
Give thanks for the mountains, rivers,
valleys and trees.
Find a moment today and fall to your
knees and kiss the earth.
Then laugh, or cry, or dance ecstatically.
Better yet, do all three.

ANCIENT WISDOM
FOR
MODERN TIMES

Ayurvedic Proverb

When diet is wrong
medicine is of no use.

When diet is correct
medicine is of no need.

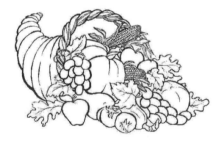

Appendix I

Ayurveda

Ayurveda, which means "the science of life," dates back five to ten thousand years, and is widely considered to be the oldest form of health care in the world. It is a holistic system of wellbeing that covers vast areas of medicine, including general practice, surgery, physiology, gynecology, psychology, pediatrics, pharmacology, herbology, tonics and rejuvenation, and sciences of the subtle body.

Over the millennia, the knowledge of Ayurveda spread out from India and influenced the ancient Chinese system of medicine, and the humoral medicine practiced by Hippocrates in Greece. For this reason, Ayurveda is often referred to as the "Mother of All Healing."

The aim of Ayurveda is vibrancy, balance, longevity, and robust health, achieved by balancing energies at all levels of being. Its centerpiece is the system of Tri-Dosha, which articulates the primary characteristics of human beings and how to bring them into balance.

This nature-based system of health springs from the native wisdom of the Vedic sages and their uncompromising adherence to the cosmic rhythms of life. The elements of nature, its natural cycles and seasons, are an integral part of this sacred science.

Ayurveda also is based upon the principle of self-knowledge. Its goal is not simply health as an end in itself, but health as a basis for self-understanding, for the recognition of our true nature and living in accord with it. From this point of view, it is not enough to treat patients from the outside. Ayurveda also seeks to aid them in self-understanding and self-unfoldment.

Ayurveda thus always aims at self-care, teaching the individual how to live in harmony with his or her own nature. This emphasis on self-knowledge, rather than on just some outer cure, is the spiritual integrity of Ayurveda.

Ayurveda & Diet

Ayurveda considers food to either be medicine or poison. A fresh, local, organic whole food, plant based diet is considered optimal. A healthy vegetarian diet is also recommended for all following the yogic path.

Processed, packaged, and junk foods are not considered to be food, but rather "foodstuff," scientifically engineered for ease of shipping, storage, and profit. These pseudo foods are a root cause of much of the illness in the world, especially in First World nations where such products are plentiful and form the basis of what is called the Western Diet. This diet is associated with the alarming rates of heart disease, cancer, diabetes, stroke, obesity, and other major diseases that are paramount in First World countries.

The practices of asana and pranayama purify the physical body. Therefore it is essential to be ingesting pure foods. Otherwise, the profoundly detoxifying and healing effect of sadhana is lost. Improper foods also affect the emotional body and contribute to stress and anxiety. Truly, therefore, we are what we eat, and our choices lead either to vibrant health or illness and diminished capacity.

Ayurveda offers detailed guidelines for "eating for your dosha." These guidelines can be invaluable for fine-tuning a yogic diet, but one should never get caught up in trying to follow general suggestions as if they were absolutes. In the yogic journey we ever want to be mindful of cultivating freedom and flexibility, not only in the body, but in all aspects of our lives. This does not imply freedom to make poor, unhealthy choices, but rather means not being rigid in beliefs that there is only one way to do things.

Just as there is no one body type or one single way to perform an asana, there is no single diet for all beings, no "one size fits all" in any aspect of yogic practice. Most importantly, when considering an Ayurvedic diet, one should seek guidance from a qualified Ayurvedic practitioner.

Dietary Overview for Vata Dosha

A nutritional program for Vata includes foods that are liquid or unctuous in your daily diet to balance dryness. Enjoy some "heavy" foods to offer substance and sustained nourishment. Foods that are smooth in texture offset roughness, foods that are warm or hot balance the cool nature of Vata.

If you need to balance Vata, a fat-free diet is not for you. Cook foods with a little ghee (clarified butter) or include some olive oil in your diet everyday. Olive oil cannot be heated to high temperatures without destroying its healing value, so drizzle olive oil over fresh soft flatbreads, cooked grains, or warm vegetable dishes. Ghee can be heated to high temperatures without affecting its nourishing, healing qualities, so use ghee to sauté vegetables, spices or other foods. Avoid too many dry foods such as crackers, dry cold cereal, and the like.

Cooked foods, served hot or warm, are ideal for balancing Vata. Pureed soups, cooked fruit, hot cereal, rice pudding, and hot nourishing beverages such as nut milks or warm milk are excellent "comfort" foods and help pacify aggravated Vata. Avoid or minimize raw foods such as salads and raw sprouts.

The three Ayurvedic tastes that help balance Vata are sweet, sour, and salty, so include more of these tastes in your daily diet. Milk, citrus fruits, fruit, or salted toasted sunflower or pumpkin seeds make good snack choices. Eat less of the bitter, pungent, or astringent tastes.

Nuts are wonderful Vata-pacifiers. Soak ten almonds overnight. Blanch and eat them in the early morning for a healthy burst of energy. Walnuts, hazelnuts, and cashews also make good Vata-pacifying snacks.

Carrots, asparagus, tender leafy greens, beets, sweet potatoes, and summer squash are the best vegetable choices. They become more digestible when chopped and cooked with Vata-pacifying spices. Vegetables can be combined with grains or mung beans for satisfying one-dish meals. Avoid nightshades and larger beans.

Basmati rice is ideal for balancing Vata. Cook it with a little salt and ghee for added flavor. Wheat is also good in the form of fresh flatbreads made with whole-wheat flour (called atta or chapatti flour and available at Indian grocery stores) and drizzled with a little melted ghee. These flatbreads combine well with cooked vegetables or Vata-balancing chutneys.

Most spices are warming and enhance digestion, so cook with a combination of spices that appeal to your taste buds and are appropriate for the dish you are making. Ayurvedic spices such as small quantities of turmeric, cumin, coriander, dried ginger, black pepper, and saffron offer flavor, aroma, and healing wisdom.

Drink plenty of warm water throughout the day.

Dietary Overview for Pitta Dosha

A nutritional program for Pitta includes a few dry foods in your daily diet to balance the liquid nature of Pitta, some "heavy" foods that offer substance and sustained nourishment, and foods that are cool to balance the fiery quality of Pitta.

If you need to balance Pitta, choose ghee (clarified butter), in moderate quantities, as your cooking medium. Ghee, according to the ancient Ayurvedic texts, is cooling for both mind and body. Ghee can be heated to high temperatures without affecting its nourishing, healing qualities, so use ghee to sauté vegetables, spices, or other foods.

Cooling foods are wonderful for balancing Pitta dosha. Sweet juicy fruits, especially pears, can cool a fiery Pitta quickly. Milk, sweet rice pudding, coconut and coconut juice, and milkshakes made with ripe mangoes and almonds or dates are examples of soothing Pitta-pacifying foods.

The three Ayurvedic tastes that help balance Pitta are sweet, bitter, and astringent, so include more of these tastes in your daily diet. Milk, fully ripe sweet fruits, and soaked or blanched almonds make good snack choices. Eat less of the salty, pungent, and sour tastes.

Dry cereal, crackers, granola, cereal bars, and rice cakes balance the liquid nature of Pitta dosha, and can be eaten any time hunger pangs strike during the day.

Carrots, asparagus, bitter leafy greens, fennel, cruciferous vegetables such as broccoli, cauliflower, and Brussels sprouts, green beans, and bitter gourd (in very small quantities) are good vegetable choices. They become more digestible when chopped and cooked with Pitta-pacifying spices. Vegetables can be combined with grains or mung beans for satisfying one-dish meals. Avoid nightshades.

Basmati rice is excellent for balancing Pitta. Wheat can also be good—fresh flatbreads made with whole wheat flour (called atta or chapatti flour and available at Indian grocery stores) combine well with cooked vegetables or Pitta-balancing chutneys. Oats and amaranth are other Pitta-balancing grains.

Choose spices that are not too heating or pungent. Ayurvedic spices such as small quantities of turmeric, cumin, coriander, cinnamon, cardamom, and fennel offer flavor, aroma and healing wisdom.

Dietary Overview for Kapha Dosha

A nutritional program for Kapha includes a few dry foods in your daily diet to balance the oily nature of Kapha. Such foods are nourishing but light. This counters the heaviness of Kapha. Warm foods with a spicy zest to them help balance the sweet, cold quality of Kapha.

If you need to balance Kapha, choose ghee (clarified butter), in very small quantities, as your cooking medium. Ghee can be heated to high temperatures without affecting its nourishing, healing qualities, so use ghee to sauté vegetables, spices or other foods. Steaming foods and then adding a mixture of spices sautéed in very little ghee is best. In general, avoid too many oily foods.

Light, warming foods help balance Kapha. Clear vegetable soups with beans and diced vegetables, stews made with Kapha-balancing vegetables, bean casseroles, dhal soups, and light grain and vegetable combinations are ideal for Kapha, especially when combined with Kapha balancing spices. Stay away from too much salt and instead infuse dishes with fresh herbs and spices for flavor.

The three Ayurvedic tastes that help balance Kapha are pungent, bitter, and astringent, so include more of these tastes in your daily diet. Apples, garbanzo beans cooked with Kapha-balancing spices, or steamed broccoli or cauliflower with a light olive oil and spice mixture make healthy Kapha-pacifying snacks. Eat less of the salty, sweet, or sour tastes.

Dry cereal, salt-free crackers, and rice cakes balance the liquid nature of Kapha dosha and make good snacks. However, eat snacks in moderation if you are trying to balance Kapha, and avoid sugary snacks. Honey in small quantities is the recommended sweetener for Kapha.

Carrots, asparagus, okra, bitter leafy greens, cruciferous vegetables such as broccoli, cauliflower, and Brussels sprouts, daikon radish and bitter gourd are good vegetable choices. They become more digestible when chopped and cooked with Kapha-pacifying spices. Vegetables can be combined with lighter grains or mung beans for satisfying one-dish meals. Avoid nightshades. Fresh green chili peppers and fresh ginger root add flavor while balancing Kapha.

Choose lighter whole grains, and eat grains in moderation. Barley, buckwheat, millet, and couscous are good choices. If you choose heavier grains such as rice or wheat, eat very small quantities.

Zesty warming spices are wonderful for balancing Kapha. Ayurvedic spices such as turmeric, cumin, coriander, cayenne, black pepper, dried ginger, asafetida (hing), cloves, and fenugreek offer flavor, aroma, and healing wisdom.

Mindfulness with Food

- Before choosing your meal ask: Do I want really this food to be a part of me? Make sure your inner wisdom knows that the food you are choosing is the best and purest possible.
- Then ask: Do I want to consume more food than I need? Don't put extra on your plate because you will feel compelled to consume it. Remind yourself that

overeating is a subtle form of greed, attachment, habit, self-centeredness, distraction, and dishonoring to your body, which is the Sacred Temple of your Spirit.

- Become deeply present with the process of preparing your meals, acknowledging your food as sacred and vital energy for body, mind, and soul.
- Drink in the visual beauty of what you are preparing, feeling deep gratitude for all the energy of nature and humankind that has made it possible for this food to arrive at your table. If you are eating out, have the same appreciation when your food is served.
- Resolve to engage in the art of dining. Light candles when possible, play soothing music, unplug the phone, turn off the TV, minimize conversation and mental wandering. Perhaps you might choose to periodically dine in complete silence, making your meal a form of meditation.
- Take time before beginning your meal to remind yourself that your body is the Temple of your Spirit and that you resolve to always honor it as such. Say a simple prayer, out loud or silently to yourself, giving deep and heartfelt thanks for this sacred nourishment.
- Before taking your first bite, pause to again drink in the beauty of your meal, noticing the rich colors and shapes. Savor the aroma deeply, breathing it into the core of your being. Take your time with each bite, chewing slowly, noticing the texture and temperature, allowing the juices and flavors to permeate your taste buds before swallowing. Once you swallow, follow the process and feel your food fully entering your body before beginning to take your next bite.
- Slow down and chew each bite a minimum of 20 times. This satisfies the body physically and

psychologically, promotes healthier digestion and provides a sense of fullness with smaller portions.
- Pause now and then, reminding yourself that you are nourishing your mind and spirit as well as your body. You and this food are becoming one, dancing together in the miraculous circle of life.

Deep Yoga Ayurvedic Food Guidelines

- Eat for your dosha as often as possible.
- Always bless your food.
- Eat slowly and mindfully.
- No TV or unnecessary conversation while dining.
- Eat often in silence.
- Eat fresh, organic food.
- Eat predominantly or completely vegetarian.
- Balance legumes, vegetables, fruits & nuts.
- No processed, canned, frozen, packaged, or junk foods.
- Do not overcook your food.
- Do not over spice your food.
- No cold drinks while dining.
- Take hot water with meals to promote digestion.
- Lunch should be your largest meal.
- Do not eat late in the evening.
- Do not eat just before bed.
- Fill the belly half with food, ¼ water, leave ¼ empty.
- Never eat when you are not truly hungry.
- Do not eat for distraction.
- Do not eat solely for taste.
- Fast regularly to allow the digestive system to purify.
- Seek to exercise after each meal, e.g., a fifteen minute walk.

Deep Yoga Gentle Fasting Program

Month One: Skip breakfast one day each week on the same day.

Month Two: Skip breakfast and lunch one day each week on the same day.

Month Three: Skip breakfast, lunch and dinner one day each week on the same day. Return to regular meals for three months, then repeat this cycle as necessary.

- Reduce food portions by ten to fifteen percent.
- Bless your food, then eat slowly with more attention to taste and texture.
- Stop when you feel three-quarters full.
- Eat organic as possible, predominantly vegetarian.
- No alcohol or coffee.
- Make lunch your biggest meal, small dinner.
- Eat in silence, no distractions.
- Avoid snacks.
- Don't eat out of habit, only when truly hungry.
- Try to take a walk after each meal, five to fifteen minutes.
- Treat your body as a Temple of Divine Spirit.

Note: Always listen to your body. Seek to perceive sensations of hunger as a natural digestive process and don't seek to satisfy every longing for food. However, no fasting program should ever cause pain or true discomfort. If you experience these, end your fast and consult a specialist.

Foods by Guna

Sattvic Foods
- Are fresh, juicy, light, unctuous, nourishing, sweet and tasty.
- Give the necessary energy to the body without taxing it.
- The foundation of higher states of consciousness.

Examples: juicy fruits, fresh vegetables that are easily digestible, fresh milk and butter, whole soaked or also sprouted beans, grains and nuts, many herbs and spices in the right combinations with other foods.

Rajasic Foods
- Are bitter, sour, salty, pungent, hot and dry.
- Increase the speed and excitement of the human organism.
- The foundation of motion, activity and pain.

Examples: foods that have been fried in oil or cooked too much or eaten in excess, specific foods and spices that are strongly exciting, coffee and other stimulants.

Tamasic Foods
- Are dry, old, decaying, distasteful and/or unpalatable.
- Consume a large amount of energy while being digested.
- Form a foundation for ignorance, doubt, and pessimism.

Examples: foods that have been strongly processed, canned, or frozen, and/or are old, stale, or incompatible with one other. All processed foods and junk foods are tamasic. They promote imbalance, illness, and disease.

Saints and sadhus can survive easily on sattvic foods alone. Those of us who "live in the world," and have to keep pace with its changes, also need rajasic energy. We should seek to keep a balance between sattvic and rajasic foods while avoiding tamasic foods without exception.

Always ask yourself: I this food serving my needs and nourishing me? Does it come from a source that is natural and organic? Was it grown or made for maximum profit, or with good health as the primary motivating factor?

Healing Meal - Kitchari:

In India, kitchari—a soupy porridge made from rice and mung beans —is considered a fasting food and is used to purify digestion and cleanse systemic toxins. It is the primary food prescribed as medicine in the practice of Ayurveda.

Ayurvedic physicians often prescribe a kitchari diet to cleanse toxins stored in bodily tissues as it restores systemic balance. Kitchari provides solid nourishment while allowing the body to devote energy to healing. You can safely subsist on kitchari anytime to build vitality and strength as it helps balance all three doshas. For restless Vata, the warm soup is grounding; for fiery Pitta, its spices are calming; and for chilly Kapha, it provides healing warmth.

Digestive Fire
Ayurveda believes that all healing begins with the digestive tract, and kitchari can give it a much-needed rest from constantly processing different foods while also providing essential nutrients. The blending of rice and split mung beans offers an array of amino acids, the building blocks of protein. Kitchari's mixture of spices enkindles the digestive fire, which is weakened by poor food combinations.

Kitchari tastes like a cross between a creamy rice cereal and a light dal, or lentil soup. If it is a cold, blustery day or you are feeling under the weather, a steaming bowl of this classic Indian comfort food can both warm up your bones and restore sagging energy.

We halve the amounts of the recipe if it is just for two people, and eat the kitchari on its own as a complete meal. Steamed vegetables add variety. Kitchari is also good with plain yogurt for excess Vata or Pitta. For excess Kapha, add cayenne to the spices and increase amounts of ginger, black pepper and cloves.

Deep Yoga Kitchari Recipe

Ingredients:
Mung Beans, split, one cup
Basmati Rice,
Cilantro, handful
Ginger, small piece peeled and chopped
Shredded Coconut
Cinnamon, Clove powder, Cardamom, Black Pepper, Turmeric, 3 Bay leaves
Salt, Asafetida (hing)

Rinse one cup of split mung beans and soak for several hours. Set aside. In a blender, liquefy one tablespoon of chopped ginger, two tablespoons of shredded coconut, and a handful of cilantro with one-half cup of water. In a large saucepan, lightly brown one-half teaspoon cinnamon; one-quarter teaspoon each of cardamom, pepper, clove powder, turmeric and three bay leaves (remove before serving) in three tablespoons of ghee, or coconut oil, or a blend of both.
Drain the mung dal and then stir it into the spice mixture in the saucepan. Next, add one cup of raw basmati rice. Stir in the blended cilantro, ginger and coconut mixture, followed by six cups of water. Bring to a boil, cover, and cook on low heat for approximately 60 minutes until soft.

Melt one tablespoon of ghee in a small saucepan. Add the salt and asafetida and stir. Sauté for one minute then add spices to mixture and serve.

For a host of delicious Ayurvedic recipes my wife, Laura Plumb, has a beautiful and highly informative blog: **www.food-alovestory.com**

Appendix II
Ayurveda Forms

Dosha Form

Determining your individual constitution, called your dosha in Ayurveda, can provide you insight into your unique nature and how to balance it to avoid mental and physical challenges. When filling out the dosha form, answer each question quickly and intuitively. Note the categories in the following form of your physical attributes, temperament, and how you usually respond to stress.

Be completely candid with yourself. Check each aspect that characterizes without over-thinking it or trying to determine what is a negative or positive reflection of you. Calculate your score in each horizontal segment for Vata, Pitta, and Kapha, then note the totals at the bottom of the chart. This will give you beginning insight into your dosha.

In its full application, the determination and analysis of doshas and imbalances is highly complex and takes into account a multiplicity of factors, including lifestyle, psychology, age, occupation, philosophy, and physiology. If you desire deeper insights into your dosha, always consult a qualified Ayurveda practitioner.

Guna Form

On the guna form, circle one the three options for each line, e.g., are you vegetarian, do you eat some meat, or do you have a heavy meat diet? When finished, add the vertical columns and total your scores for Sattva, Rajas, and Tamas.

As you continue your journey of moving towards greater wellness, seek to shift all aspects of your life towards the Sattva column. Again, go slowly. Be gentle with yourself. Don't try to seek perfection or you are likely to set yourself up for failure and lowered self-esteem. Small shifts, sustained over time, however, become great victories and help you move forward on your healing journey.

Deep Yoga Dosha Form

Physical		Temperament		Under Stress		
Thin Frame	__	Talks Fast, A Lot	__	Weight Loss	__	
Prominent Joints	__	Indecisive	__	Constipation	__	
Very Tall or Short	__	Learns Fast/Forgets	__	Excess Gas	__	**V**
Variable Appetite	__	Enthusiastic/Joyful	__	Restless/Active	__	**A**
Weight at Middle	__	Psychic	__	Chronic Pain	__	**T**
Chilly	__	Sensitive to Noise	__	Light Sleep	__	**A**
Dry, Kinky Hair	__	Creative/Artistic	__	Anxious/Fearful	__	
Small, Dry Eyes	__	Intuitive	__	Variable Energy	__	
Joint Discomfort	__	Introspective	__	Panic Attacks	__	
Physical		**Temperament**		**Under Stress**		
Medium Build	__	Sharp/Concise	__	Rashes	__	
Athletic	__	Competitive	__	Excess Sweat	__	
Warm-Blooded	__	Intelligent/Perceptive	__	Body Odor	__	**P**
Oily, Soft Skin	__	Keen Memory	__	Gastritis/Ulcers	__	**I**
Freckles/Pimples	__	Irritable/Impatient	__	High Blood Pressure	__	**T**
Premature Grey	__	Successful	__	Short Sleep	__	**T**
Straight, Fine Hair	__	Jealous	__	Likes Hot Spices	__	**A**
Pink, Pliable Nails	__	Courageous	__	Alcohol to Excess	__	
Undue Hunger	__	Organized/Efficient	__	Anger/Violent	__	
Physical		**Temperament**		**Under Stress**		
Thick, Wide Frame	__	Slow Speech	__	Oversleep	__	
Good Stamina	__	Calm	__	Overeat	__	
Strong	__	Responsible	__	Loss of Appetite	__	**K**
Thick, Oily Skin	__	Steady Faith	__	Excess Mucus	__	**A**
Weight in Hips	__	Long Memory	__	Water Retention	__	**P**
White, Even Teeth	__	Stubborn	__	Laziness	__	**H**
Thick, Lustrous Hair	__	Forgiving	__	Inactive	__	**A**
Large Eyes	__	Loyal	__	Greedy	__	
Lubricated Joints	__	Nurturing	__	Depressed	__	

Your Dosha Score: Vata_____ Pitta_____ Kapha_____

Deep Yoga Guna Form

	Sattva	Rajas	Tamas
DIET:	Vegetarian	Some Meat	Heavy Meat Diet
DRUGS/ALCOHOL:	Never	Occasionally	Frequently
NEED FOR SLEEP:	Little	Moderate	High
SEXUAL ACTIVITY:	Little	Moderate	High
IN NATURE:	Frequently	Occasionally	Never
CONTROL OF SENSES:	Good	Moderate	Weak
SPEECH:	Calm, Peaceful	Agitated	Dull
WORK:	Selfless	Personal Gain	Lazy
ANGER:	Rarely	Sometimes	Frequently
VIOLENT BEHAVIOR:	Never	Sometimes	Frequent
FEAR:	Rarely	Sometimes	Frequently
DESIRE:	Little	Some	A Lot
ATTACHMENT TO MONEY:	Little	Some	A Lot
PRIDE:	Modest	Some Ego	Vain
DEPRESSION:	Never	Sometimes	Frequent
LOVE:	Universal	Personal	Lacking
CONTENTMENT:	Usually	Partly	Never
FORGIVENESS:	Forgives Easily	With Effort	Hold Grudges
CONCENTRATION:	Good	Moderate	Poor
MEMORY:	Good	Moderate	Poor
WILLPOWER:	Strong	Variable	Weak
TRUTHFULNESS:	Always	Mostly	Rarely
PEACE OF MIND:	Generally	Partly	Rarely
CREATIVITY:	High	Moderate	Low
SPIRITUAL STUDY:	Daily	Occasionally	Never
MANTRA, PRAYER:	Daily	Occasionally	Never
MEDITATION:	Daily	Occasionally	Never
ASANA/PRANAYAMA:	Daily	Occasionally	Never
SERVICE:	Often	Some	None

Your Guna Score: Tamas_____ Rajas_____ Sattva_____

Appendix III
Sanskrit Glossary

Abhinivesha: Fear of our ego not being able to control reality
Abhyasa: Perseverance, commitment to practice
Aham Brahmasmi: I and the Divine are one
Agama: Knowledge gained through reading sacred texts
Ahamkara: Sense of I-ness, ego
Ahimsa: Non-harming, nonviolence
Ajna: Sixth chakra
Anahata: Fourth chakra
Anjali Mudra: Palms brought together at the heart center
Anumana: Knowledge through inference
Aparigraha: Non-possessiveness
Asana: Yoga postures; third limb in Patanjali's Eight Limbs of Yoga
Ashtanga: Eight Limbs; refers to Pantanjali's system of Yoga in the Yoga Sutras
Asmita: Identifying ourselves through the ego
Asteya: Non-stealing
Atman: The soul, the deeper self
Avidya: Lack of wisdom, ignorance of who we truly are
Ayurveda: Medical system of Yoga; "Science of Life"
Bhagavad-Gita: A sacred text of yogic spirituality
Bhakti: Yoga path of devotion
Bramacharya: Not overindulging the sense
Buddhi: Intuitive intelligence, wisdom, the "higher mind"
Chakra: An energy vortex in the subtle body
Dharana: Concentration; sixth limb of Patanjali's Eight Limbs of Yoga
Dharma: Universal Law; one's individual true path in life
Dhyana: Meditation; seventh limb in Patanjali's Eight Limbs of Yoga
Dosha: An imbalance; an aspect of the human constitution
Dukkha: Suffering, affliction, pain, anxiety
Dvesha: Aversion to challenging experiences, dislikes

Granthis: Psychic knots.
Gunas: Qualities or attributes of life
Guru: Teacher, darkness to light
Hatha: Yoga of purification
Ishvara: The Divine, God, Higher Power
Ishvara Pranidhana: Constant awareness of the Divine
Jivanmukti: Liberated being
Jnana: Yoga path of wisdom
Jyotish: Astrological system of Yoga
Kapha: One of the three doshas; related to the elements of water and earth
Karma: The cycle of cause and effect
Kleshas: Mental states that cloud our true nature and create suffering
Mahabhutas: The five elements of earth, water, fire, air, and space
Mahat: Cosmic intelligence
Manas: Lower mind
Manipura: Third chakra
Mantra: Spiritual poems or phrases usually repeated or chanted
Mauna: Silence, pure awareness.
Moksha: Liberation
Muladhara: First chakra
Namaste: Indian greeting or parting phrase; "From the light in my heart, I bow to the light in your heart"
Niyamas: Personal observances; second limb in Patanjali's Eight Limbs of Yoga
OM Tat Sat: I am That
Pitta: One of the three Doshas; related to the element of fire
Prajna: Flashes of illumination.
Prakriti: the basic matter of which the universe consists
Pramana: Right knowledge
Prana: Life force
Pranayama: Control of and mastery of the life force
Prasadanam: Undisturbed calmness.
Pratipaksha Bhavana: Cultivation of an opposite emotion

Pratyahara: Withdrawal of the senses; fifth limb in Patanjali's Eight Limbs of Yoga

Pratyaksha: Knowledge gained through direct experience

Purusha: The soul, Atman

Raga: Attraction to our perceived pleasures

Raja Yoga: Royal path of Yoga

Rajas: One of the three Gunas; associated with activity

Rishi: Sage

Sadhana: Daily spiritual practice

Sahashara: Seventh chakra

Samadhi: Absorption, enlightenment; eighth limb of Patanjali's Eight Limbs of Yoga

Samkalpa: A positive resolve

Samskara: Deep-seated impressions that create habituated responses to life

Santosha: Contentment

Satchitananda: Being, consciousness, and bliss

Satsang: Students gathering before a teacher for lessons in Yogic philosophy

Sattva: One of the three Gunas; associated with balance and equilibrium

Satya: Truthfulness

Saucha: Purity

Savasana: Corpse pose

Shanti: Peace

Shrada: Faith

Smriti: Remembering the insights that arise during your contemplations and practices.

Svadhyaya: Spiritual studies, self-inquiry

Swadhisthana: Second chakra

Tamas: One of the three Gunas; associated with darkness and inertia

Tapas: Sustained self-discipline

Tridosha: Ayurveda system of Three Doshas

Vairagya: Detachment from outcomes

Vata: One of the three doshas; related to the element of air

Vedanta: Indian philosophy dealing with the reality of nature
Vidya: Eternal and innate wisdom.
Vikalpa: False information
Vinyasa: Flowing series of Yoga poses
Viparaya: Delusion
Vishuddhi: Fifth chakra
Viveka: Discernment. Conscious choices.
Vedas: Ancient spiritual texts from which Yoga and Ayurveda arose
Virya: Courage
Yamas: Moral precepts; first limb in Patanjali's Eight Limbs of Yoga
Yoga Sutras: Aphorisms of Yoga practice by the sage Patanjali

About the Author

Bhava Ram (Brad Willis) is the cofounder of the Deep Yoga School of Healing Arts™, a system of yogic art and science blending ancient techniques of Vedanta, Yoga, and Ayurveda. Ram leads retreats, workshops, and seminars worldwide, and guides individual clients in mind/body healing, meditation, Yoga, spiritual awakening. He has served as faculty for *Yoga Journal* conferences, the International Yoga Festival in Rishikesh, India, the Omega Institute, and the Kripalu Center for Yoga and Health.

Previously, Ram worked and lived and worked throughout much of the world as a network news foreign correspondent covering many of the most momentous events of our times. A broken back and failed surgery crippled and disabled Ram, forcing him into early retirement. Subsequently, a rare and fatal form of cancer, most likely contracted while covering the Persian Gulf War, spread throughout his body. On the brink of death, he embraced Yoga in all of its aspects, fully devoting his life to studying and practicing mind/body medicine, self-healing and personal transformation. This journey led to overcoming constant pain, and ultimately healing from stage four cancer. Ram is now devoted to sharing the message that we all have the capacity to take charge of our lives, heal ourselves, and reach profound levels of physical, emotional and spiritual well-being.

Ram is certified as an Advanced Yoga & Ayurveda Educator through the American Institute of Vedic Studies and as an Ayurvedic Wellness Counselor through the Kerala Ayurveda Academy of India. He registered as a Yoga Instructor through the Yoga Alliance at the highest, ERYT 500-hour level. Deep Yoga is registered as a 200 and 500 hour teaching school through the Yoga Alliance.

Through Deep Yoga, Bhava Ram also contributes to charitable projects for at risk youth and disabled children.

Also by Bhava Ram

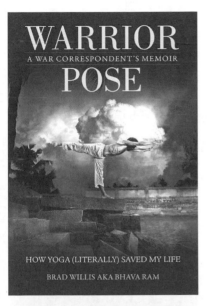

**Warrior Pose:
How Yoga (Literally) Saved My Life**
Bhava Ram's highly acclaimed memoir of life as a war correspondent, facing a broken back and stage four cancer, and healing through Yoga and Ayurveda. 2013

"Warrior Pose is Indiana Jones merged with Gautama Buddha, a miraculous affirmation of the power of self-healing, a war story, a love story, and a spiritual journey of epic proportion..."

Dr. Emmett Miller
Pioneer of Mind/Body Medicine

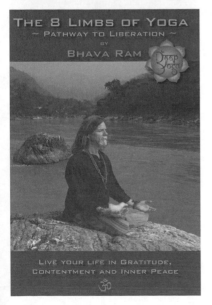

**The Eight Limbs of Yoga:
Pathway to Liberation**
Bhava Ram explores the centerpiece of Raja Yoga known as Ashtanga, or the Eight Limbs and provides practices so that we can incorporate this time-tested wisdom into our daily lives. 2009

"Bhava's style and down to earth explanations really opened my understanding to the true power that Yoga can have in a person's life."

Dr. Adam Meyerowitz

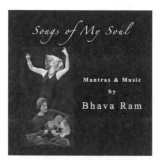

Songs of My Soul CD (iTunes & CD Baby)

Bhava Ram's latest album in collaboration with performing artist Hans Christian.

"Bhava's devotion, unique compositions, expressive voice and wide open heart make his music an uplifting and unforgettable experience." Sundaram, Jyoti Mandir

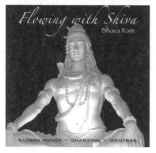

Flowing With Shiva CD (iTunes & CD Baby)

Bhava Ram's first album of devotional music, composed in Rishikesh, India. Each piece blends Sanskrit mantras with English lyrics and interpretations to create a spiritual meditation through sacred sound.

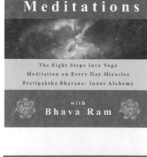

Meditation CD (iTunes & CD Baby)

Three meditation practices. Experience the Eight Steps Into Yoga, Meditation on Miracles, and Pratipaksha Bhavana.

These meditations are designed to bring you into states of deeper inner awareness, cultivate a richer awareness of the miracles of life, and shift your inner chemistry.

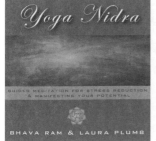

Yoga Nidra CD (www.deepyoga.com)

Yoga Nidra promotes profound relaxation, healing and inner peace while supporting new behaviors and personal growth.

Recorded by Bhava Ram & Laura Plumb.

Booking Lectures, Workshops, Trainings

Bhava Ram gives keynote speeches, workshops, and lectures for medical conferences and corporate venues.

He provides experiential workshops at Yoga Studios, Retreat Centers, and in educational forums.

Ram also consults with private clients in person, or via telephone, Skype, and Face Time.

To book Bhava Ram as a speaker or
schedule private sessions please contact:

info@deepyoga.com

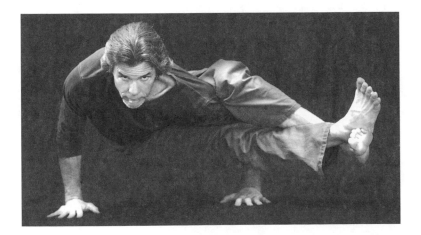

For more on Bhava Ram and Deep Yoga please see:

deepyoga.com
and
bhavaram.com

ANCIENT WISDOM
FOR
MODERN TIMES

Yoga

Yoga is living fully
in the present moment.

Yoga is unifying
with the inner wisdom of your Soul.

Yoga is realizing the
oneness of all that is.

Yoga is the journey home
to who you always have been.